Diversity & Cultural Awareness in Nursing Practice

Diversity & Cultural Awareness in Nursing Practice

Edited by
Beverley Brathwaite

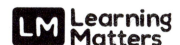
LM Learning Matters

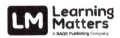

Learning Matters
A SAGE Publishing Company
1 Oliver's Yard
55 City Road
London EC1Y 1SP

SAGE Publications Inc.
2455 Teller Road
Thousand Oaks, California 91320

SAGE Publications India Pvt Ltd
B 1/I 1 Mohan Cooperative Industrial Area
Mathura Road
New Delhi 110 044

SAGE Publications Asia-Pacific Pte Ltd
3 Church Street
#10-04 Samsung Hub
Singapore 049483

Editor: Donna Goddard
Development editor: Eleanor Rivers
Senior project editor: Chris Marke
Project management: Swales & Willis Ltd, Exeter, Devon
Marketing manager: George Kimble
Cover design: Wendy Scott
Typeset by: C&M Digitals (P) Ltd, Chennai, India
Printed in the UK

Library of Congress Control Number: 2019948795

British Library Cataloguing in Publication Data

A catalogue record for this book is available from the British Library

ISBN 978-1-5264-2433-4
ISBN 978-1-5264-2434-1 (pbk)

At SAGE we take sustainability seriously. Most of our products are printed in the UK using responsibly sourced papers and boards. When we print overseas we ensure sustainable papers are used as measured by the PREPS grading system. We undertake an annual audit to monitor our sustainability.

Contents

About the authors   viii

Introduction   1
Beverley Brathwaite

1   Diversity, health inequality and nursing   6
     Beverley Brathwaite

2   Diversity and cultural concepts of health   21
     Beverley Brathwaite

3   Diversity, communication and health literacy   43
     Marion Hinds

4   Cultural competency   69
     Marion Hinds

5   Assessing the needs of diverse patients   94
     Mariama Seray-Wurie and Beverley Brathwaite

6   Spirituality, death, grief and loss   112
     Beverley Brathwaite

7   Public health: meeting the needs of diverse communities   129
     Gillian Craig and Caroline McGraw

8   Mental distress and cultural diversity   154
     Nicky Lambert

References   172
Index   200

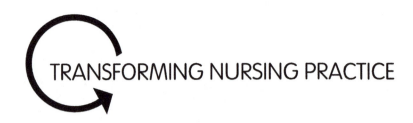

TRANSFORMING NURSING PRACTICE

Transforming Nursing Practice is a series tailor made for pre-registration students nurses. Each book in the series is:

 Affordable

 Mapped to the NMC Standards of proficiency for registered nurses

 Full of active learning features

 Focused on applying theory to practice

Each book addresses a core topic and they have been carefully developed to be simple to use, quick to read and written in clear language.

An invaluable series of books that explicitly relates to the NMC standards. Each book covers a different topic that students need to explore in order to develop into a qualified nurse... I would recommend this series to all Pre-Registered nursing students whatever their field or year of study.

LINDA ROBSON,
Senior Lecturer at Edge Hill University

Many titles in the series are on our recommended reading list and for good reason - the content is up to date and easy to read. These are the books that actually get used beyond training and into your nursing career.

EMMA LYDON,
Adult Student Nursing

ABOUT THE SERIES EDITORS

DR MOOI STANDING is an Independent Academic Nursing Consultant (UK and international) responsible for the core knowledge, personal and professional learning skills titles. She has invaluable experience as an NMC Quality Assurance Reviewer of educational programmes, and as a Professional Regulator Panellist on the NMC Practice Committee. Mooi is also a Board member of Special Olympics Malaysia.

DR SANDRA WALKER is a Clinical Academic in Mental Health working between North Bristol Trust and Southern Health Trust. She is series editor for the mental health nursing titles. She is a Qualified Mental Health Nurse with a wide range of clinical experience spanning 30 years and spent several years working as a mental health lecturer at Southampton University.

BESTSELLING TEXTBOOKS

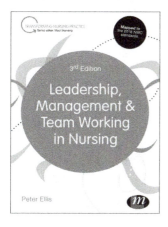

3rd Edition

Leadership, Management & Team Working in Nursing

Peter Ellis

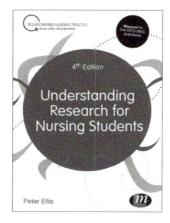

4th Edition

Understanding Research for Nursing Students

Peter Ellis

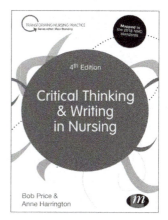

4th Edition

Critical Thinking & Writing in Nursing

Bob Price & Anne Harrington

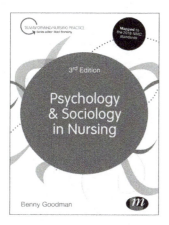

3rd Edition

Psychology & Sociology in Nursing

Benny Goodman

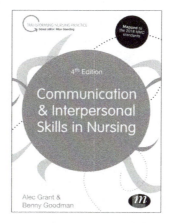

4th Edition

Communication & Interpersonal Skills in Nursing

Alec Grant & Benny Goodman

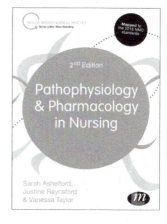

2nd Edition

Pathophysiology & Pharmacology in Nursing

Sarah Ashelford, Justine Raynsford & Vanessa Taylor

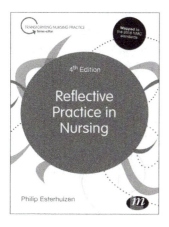

4th Edition

Reflective Practice in Nursing

Philip Esterhuizen

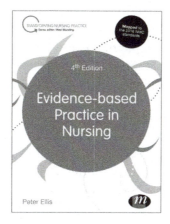

4th Edition

Evidence-based Practice in Nursing

Peter Ellis

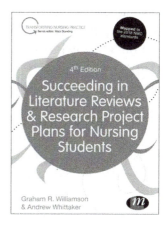

4th Edition

Succeeding in Literature Reviews & Research Project Plans for Nursing Students

Graham R. Williamson & Andrew Whittaker

You can find a full list of textbooks in the
Transforming Nursing Practice series at
https://uk.sagepub.com

About the authors

Beverley Brathwaite became a registered adult nurse in 1991, working clinically in acute general medicine, tissue viability and practice development. Gaining a degree and MSc, Beverley is also a registered teacher with the NMC and currently working on her PhD. Beverley's teaching focus has ranged from tissue viability, to acute and long-term nursing care, to evidence-based practice, to inequalities in health. She has worked with undergraduate degree students from all fields, as well as nursing associates.

Gillian Craig specialises in public health and social science, and has a particular interest in inclusion health and social diversity. Her research areas include supportive models of practice for marginalised groups with tuberculosis, and maternal feeding practices and children with neurodisability. She has recently completed an NIHR-funded project on models of psychosocial support for children with neurodisability and complex feeding needs and their families. She has co-authored several chapters in the *Tuberculosis Stigma Measurement Guidance* developed by the USAID-funded, KNCV-led Challenge TB project. She holds an honorary position with City, University of London.

Marion Hinds is a senior lecturer in adult nursing at Middlesex University with over 35 years of clinical nursing experience in intensive and high-dependency nursing. She has an MA in policy organisation and change in professional care, and is a registered nurse teacher with the NMC. Academic experience includes lecturing on pre-registration and post-registration programmes. She has a particular interest in the theory and practice of the nursing process and care planning, and is co-chair of a biannual care planning conference for nursing students. Marion has also presented at UK and international conferences on the use of the viva as an effective assessment tool for nursing students.

Nicky Lambert is an associate professor (practice) at Middlesex University, where she is Director of Teaching and Learning for Mental Health, Social Work and Integrative Medicine. She is registered as a specialist practitioner (NMC) and is a senior teaching fellow (SFHEA). Nicky has worked across a range of mental health services both in the UK and internationally, supporting staff and practice development in acute and mental health trusts, councils, businesses and charities. She is also a specialist advisor on women's well-being, mental health and nurse education. She is a community activist, a researcher and a trustee for a women's centre.

Caroline McGraw is a registered nurse, specialist practitioner qualification district nurse and qualified teacher. She is currently a lecturer in the School of Health Sciences at City, University of London and programme director for the undergraduate health and social care programme. Caroline's past clinical roles include lead district nurse for education and training, professional development district nurse, partnership nurse for victims of crime and district nurse team leader. Her research interests focus on risk management in home healthcare settings.

Mariama Seray-Wurie became a registered adult nurse in 1990 and has been a lecturer at the University of West London and a senior lecturer in adult nursing at Middlesex University since 2005. Her clinical background was in infectious diseases and haematology, and she graduated with an MA in Learning and Teaching in Healthcare in 2005 and is a registered teacher with the NMC. Mariama's teaching focus is mainly with pre-registration nursing curriculum development and programme management as the Director of Programmes for Adult Nursing at Middlesex University, acute nursing care, clinical skills and simulated practice learning. She has also presented at national and international conferences on student experiences.

Introduction

Beverley Brathwaite

Who is this book for?

This book is aimed at undergraduate pre-registration nursing students and nursing associates who will complete their programmes and register with the Nursing and Midwifery Council (NMC). The NMC has clearly identified the importance of student nurses being able to deliver care to diverse patient groups.

The role of the nurse in the twenty-first century

Registered nurses provide leadership in the delivery of care for people of all ages and from different backgrounds, cultures and beliefs. They provide nursing care for people who have complex mental, physical, cognitive and behavioural care needs, those living with dementia, the elderly, and for people at the end of their life (NMC, 2018, p3).

The main areas of this book cover generic aspects of knowledge, skills and attributes that are vital to learning about healthcare from a diversity and cultural perspective. These skills and attributes will be valuable to students of all fields of nursing and midwifery. The NMC Standards of Proficiency for Registered Nurses (NMC, 2018) is the framework on which the book is based. As with all the titles in the Transforming Nursing Practice series, the content of this book is useful for anyone who is studying to become a healthcare professional.

Why *Diversity and Cultural Awareness in Nursing Practice*?

Our patients are individual members of society who come from diverse ethnic, cultural and religious backgrounds from all over the world. Their reasons for being in the UK are equally as diverse, whether they are searching for a better quality of life and financial security, or escaping from war, terrorism and fear of persecution in their homeland. Patients/service users bring their personal cultural and religious beliefs and customs with them. It must be remembered that throughout history, British society has been, and continues to be, heavily influenced by these cultures, religions and ethnicities (EHRC, 2016b).

Members of these groups can be marginalised from society because of their differences from the majority of the population in the UK. There are other groups that can also be marginalised, such as the lesbian, gay, bisexual, transgender and queer (LGBTQ) community, patients who have mental health issues or learning disabilities, those who are physically disabled, and gypsy, Roma and traveller communities. Multidimensional perspectives on diversity will be a theme running through this book.

The following ideal should be a basic tenet of all who are and seek to be healthcare professionals: the respect of the common rights that all patients have without discrimination, and the provision of care that acknowledges, understands and appreciates patients' differences and works on addressing the barriers that patients face to deliver the right level of care for all (Baillie & Matiti, 2013).

Book structure

Chapter 1 defines the terminology and concepts that are fundamental to using this book and working with the diversity of patients who we meet as healthcare professionals. Health and inequality and equity will be examined, which will provide insight into the attitudes often held by healthcare professionals when it comes to diverse communities and care delivery.

Chapter 2 presents a broader social perspective on certain diverse groups, and considers what this has meant, and continues to mean, for their health and the delivery of care to an ever-changing population and the NHS. Concepts of social and health determinants will be expanded upon, as well as an explanation of behaviour towards access, treatment and the attitudes of diverse communities to health. Unconscious bias, stigmatisation and stereotyping will be used to demonstrate how significantly these influence care delivery to diverse patients.

Chapter 3 considers the crucial role of good communication in all its forms for providing effective care and ensuring good access to care for diverse groups. The evidence that defines and supports the rise in importance of health literacy will be examined and related to the impact that poor health literacy can have on health and illness. Effective communication is the cornerstone of patient care for all fields of nursing and HCP students. It is one of the ways in which compassion and sensitivity can be conveyed to promote collaboration and cooperation in the clinical setting. Compassion in Practice (Department of Health, 2012a), specified by the Chief Nursing Officer's 6 Cs, highlights the importance of communication and compassion. Nowhere is this more crucial than when working with diverse patient groups.

Chapter 4 argues that an understanding of the concepts of cultural competency in relation to nursing practice is a necessary prerequisite to the delivery of appropriate, effective and holistic nursing care. Before the notion of cultural competency can be understood, culture and competency must be understood as separate terms. This chapter critically discusses these two concepts. The key elements of cultural competence (awareness, sensitivity, attitudes, knowledge and skills) are then examined. Following on from this, the varied theories of cultural concepts are discussed and analysed. This will allow students to understand the complex nature of cultural competency.

A significant part of the nurse's role involves assessment and implementation of care for patients/clients, which can occur in a variety of healthcare settings. Chapter 5 explores the role of supporting and working with individuals and families from a diverse range of backgrounds, religions, cultures, ethnicities and disabilities, as well as from the LGBTQ community, which can influence how the individual perceives health and illness and how they may want to receive care.

Chapter 6 considers the definitions and theories of spirituality within diverse groups and how the nurse/student can assess the spirituality of patients in order to care for this 'hidden' need. The chapter will also show the reader how to manage their own beliefs of spirituality within the patient–nurse relationship and manage situations where their beliefs contrast with those of their patients. Healthcare professionals deal with death, grief and loss (DGL). Diverse groups approach DGL in differing ways based on cultural and religious beliefs. Identifying needs through these differing approaches should allow culturally and religiously sensitive support to be given when delivering nursing care.

Chapter 7 offers nurses an understanding of where to begin to meet the public health needs of Britain's diverse populations in the community/primary care setting. It will begin with an examination of the national policy background on public health using varied examples related to either a communicable or a non-communicable condition. It then progresses to epidemiological databases used to identify prevalence, incidence and trends related to a topical health issue to aid care delivery.

Chapter 8 argues that mental health issues are as important as physical health issues. Healthcare is delivered within a societal framework and it is important for us to understand the ways that best mental health practice can improve patients' lives. By appreciating these issues, we can explore ways for all healthcare professionals to work together and engage in delivering the best care possible for mental health service users.

Requirements for the NMC Standards of Proficiency for Registered Nurses and the proficiencies and platforms

The NMC has established standards of proficiencies of practice to be met by applicants to different parts of the register, and these are the standards it considers necessary for safe and effective practice. In addition to the standards, the NMC has set out specific proficiencies that nursing students must be able to perform at various points of an education programme. These are known as 'platforms'. This book is structured so that it will help you to understand and meet the standards and proficiencies required for entry to the NMC register. The relevant proficiencies and platforms are presented at the start of each chapter so that you can clearly see which ones the chapter addresses. There are *generic standards* that all nursing students, irrespective of their field, must achieve, and *field-specific standards* relating to each field of nursing (i.e. mental health, children's, learning disability and adult nursing).

This book includes the latest standards of proficiency for registered nursing (NMC, 2018).

Learning features

Learning by reading text is not always easy. Therefore, to provide variety and to assist with the development of independent learning skills and the application of theory to practice, this book contains activities, case studies, scenarios, further reading, useful websites and other materials to enable you to participate in your own learning. You will need to develop your own study skills and 'learn how to learn' to get the best from the material. The book cannot provide all the answers, but instead provides a framework for your learning.

The activities in the book will in particular help you to make sense of, and learn about, the material being presented. Some activities ask you to reflect on aspects of practice, or your experience of it, or the people or situations you encounter. *Reflection* is an essential skill in nursing, and it helps you to understand the world around you and often to identify how things might be improved. Other activities will help you to develop key graduate skills, such as your ability to *think critically* about a topic in order to challenge received wisdom, or your ability to *research a topic and find appropriate information and evidence*, and to be able to *make decisions* using that evidence in situations that are often difficult and time-pressured. Communication and working as part of a team are core to all nursing practice, and some activities will ask you to carry out *teamwork activities* or think about your *communication skills* to help develop these. Finally, as a registered nurse, you will be expected to *lead and manage* your own team, case load or area of care, and so some activities focus on helping you build confidence in doing this.

All the activities require you to take a break from reading the text, think through the issues presented and carry out some independent study, possibly using the internet. Where appropriate, there are sample answers presented at the end of each chapter, and these will help you to understand more fully your own reflections and independent study. Remember, academic study will always require independent work; attending lectures will never be enough to be successful on your programme, and these activities will help to deepen your knowledge and understanding of the issues under scrutiny and give you practice at working on your own.

You might want to think about completing these activities as part of your personal development plan (PDP) or portfolio. After completing an activity, write it up in your PDP or portfolio in a section devoted to that particular platform, then look back over time to see how far you are developing. You can also do more of the activities for a key skill in which you have identified a weakness, which will help build your skill and confidence in this area.

This book covers some challenging areas of society, such as racism, discrimination, inequalities in health, and how influential these issues are in giving holistic care to patients. We hope that the book allows you to think not only about how you give care, but to whom, and the social context in which our patients live and healthcare delivery takes place.

Chapter 1

Diversity, health inequality and nursing

Beverley Brathwaite

NMC Standards of Proficiency for Registered Nurses

This chapter will address the following platforms and proficiencies:

Platform 1: Being an accountable professional

1.14 provide and promote non-discriminatory, person-centred and sensitive care at all times, reflecting on people's values and beliefs, diverse backgrounds, cultural characteristics, language requirements, needs and preferences, taking account of any need for adjustments.

Platform 2: Promoting health and preventing ill health

2.3 understand the factors that may lead to inequalities in health outcomes.

Platform 7: Coordinating care

7.9 facilitate equitable access to healthcare for people who are vulnerable or have a disability, demonstrate the ability to advocate on their behalf when required, and make necessary reasonable adjustments to the assessment, planning and delivery of their care.

Chapter aims

After reading this chapter, you will be able to:

- understand the definitions of key terms used in the book;
- have an awareness of the multiple causes of inequality in healthcare within a diverse context;
- know the difference between equity and equality; and
- consider the difference between equity and equality and how this affects healthcare practice, as well as what to consider as a student nurse in order to make unbiased clinical decisions.

Introduction

Case study: Cunningham Street

In many streets in the UK, people of differing ethnic origins, faiths, religions and sexualities are living out their lives. At no. 35 Cunningham Street, Anish is of Asian descent. He has Type 2 diabetes and chronic kidney disease and is going to see his GP. At no. 12, Karen is worried about her wife having postnatal depression since the birth of their baby six months ago and has had a conversation about this with the health visitor. At no. 2, Olufunke is of Nigerian descent and has just recently been discharged from hospital following an admission due to her systemic lupus erythematosus (SLE). At no. 5, Jennifer is a young woman of Caribbean descent who is on the autistic spectrum and is waiting for an ambulance to take her to hospital with a suspected fractured ankle.

All the residents on Cunningham Street have come into contact with the NHS and healthcare professionals. They expect and deserve to be treated with an awareness and understanding of their particular needs and the world in which they live. As healthcare professionals, we must acknowledge that these persons come in contact with us as healthcare professionals in conjunction with an illness, disease or trauma that may be acute, long-term, physical or emotional, and it is our responsibility to respond to this professionally and holistically. The 6 Cs of care, compassion, competence, communication, courage and commitment (NHS England, 2015) – as well as a 7th C, consistency, to assure that the 6 Cs are performed with every healthcare encounter – is an essential part of assuring that care delivery meets the requirements of patients. Nursing knowledge that embraces all aspects of diversity and culture is imperative when carrying out safe care for all patients (Underwood, 2006).

In Chapter 1, we look at diversity and 'inequality challenges', and how important it is that you understand the inequalities and determinants of health so that equitable and individualised care can be given. It demonstrates how issues of diversity are a key component of health inequality and they must be considered carefully when planning equitable service provision. Data from the Office for National Statistics (ONS) are used to illustrate how the population has become more diverse, as well as highlighting vulnerable groups in society and in healthcare.

This chapter will show how diversity has changed in modern Britain. It will take a more detailed look at race, ethnicity and culture, and consider the importance of prejudice, stereotyping, racism, difference and unconscious bias in relation to healthcare delivery. It will also consider the inequality this promotes and how equity and equality differ. Finally, intersectionality as a concept within health, as well as its importance in acknowledging that our patients can be treated unfairly based on multiple diverse group membership, is also discussed.

There are a number of terms, such as ethnicity, culture and stereotyping, that will be used throughout the book. Although we hear and use some of these terms all the time, we do not always appreciate the complexities of their meanings. The terms in this section can only be briefly defined here. Please see the further reading section at the end of the chapter for guidance on exploring these terms in more depth.

Diversity

The term 'diversity' is a standard, mainstream term, used in a wide range of health research settings.

(Bradby and Brand, 2016, p3)

Diversity is defined as 'making sure that we recognise, respect, value and celebrate the differences that everyone has, as well as leveraging the opportunities that different people bring to the work that we do' (Health Education England, 2018, p8). These differences can be seen through the inhabitants of our street in the above case study. They can be based on ethnicity, sexual orientation, mental health issues or learning disabilities. This shows just how multifaceted and complex diversity is. Indeed, these differences or categories are only a few of many. Others include asylum seeker, immigrant, and lesbian, gay, bisexual, transgender and queer (LGBTQ), and are just that – categories – our patients are not 'simply' categories or groups. Patients/service users are fluid in how they identify themselves (Wessendorf, 2014).

Diversity is often characterised negatively by the media and parts of society, particularly when referring to topics surrounding ethnicity, immigration, asylum seekers and refugees (Vertovec, 2011; Wessendorf, 2014). Riots have erupted because of disadvantages and inequality faced by some black, Asian and minority ethnic (BAME) groups and religious and cultural groups within some sectors of society, such as education, the criminal justice system and healthcare (EHRC, 2016b). However, a central tenet of this book is that diversity is a positive feature of modern society (Wessendorf, 2014).

What is super-diversity?

Super-diversity is understood here as a lens to describe an exceptional demographic situation characterised by the multiplication of social categories within specific localities (Wessendorf, 2014).

The increasing numbers of varied groups among the population in modern Britain is based not only on ethnicity, but cultural, religious and linguistic differences. There are people who have come to the UK over the last 20 years who phenotypically look the same as the white British population but are from all over Europe. There are others with more observable physical signs of difference, such as skin colour (non-white), dress, and cultural and religious differences. These groups have a different relationship with Britain's past interactions with immigration. Black African/Caribbean and South Asian groups came to Britain by immigrating, many being British citizens from British colonies with British passports. New movements into Britain from the European Union and refugees and asylum seekers from war-torn parts of the world have generated another layer of difference not only based on skin colour, but 'new' cultural and religious differences.

Race, ethnicity and culture

Culture, race and ethnicity are terms commonly used in healthcare literature, society and clinical practice. These terms will be recurring throughout the book and, like diversity, are complex concepts with social, political, ideological and sociological differences in meanings and emphases.

The term 'race' generally refers to a social group or person appearing to have observable differing characteristics, such as skin colour, facial features and body shapes (Garner, 2017). This is breaking down multiple theories of race to its most simplistic form. However, when talking about race, it is never a simple task:

- *'Race' in biological terms (of simply what people look like) matters a lot. For example, it bears importantly on the way resources are made more or less accessible.*
- *It is not individuals alone, but also important institutions like the State, who have input in determining the meaning of 'race'.*
- *Different social systems and their cultures attach different types of meaning to physical appearance.*

(Garner, 2017, p5)

The concept of ethnicity is another way of thinking about human diversity (Dein, 2006, p69). Ethnicity refers to the importance of a collective culture that is integral to being a member of a social group and a person in this group. The focus is less on the physical attributes connected to race, but on the social grounds of shared traditions and heritage (Murji and Solomos, 2015).

Culture is a set of beliefs and practices that can be religion, dress, food, customs or music connecting people and individuals together (Parekh, 2000). Another way of looking at culture is the sharing of meanings within a given experience that comes from being a part of a group with a set of beliefs and customs. There is also a psychosocial aspect of culture concerned with 'feelings, attachments and emotions' (Hall, 1997, p2). To deliver effective care, healthcare professionals need to understand about the cultural attachments of our patients, to friends, family and other members of the wider community that share both ethnicity and culture.

As can be seen here, there are overlapping ideas of what race, ethnicity and culture mean, and this is a theoretical and political debate that carries on today (Murji and

Solomos, 2015). An important point to consider is that these are terms that are used to signify difference within society from the biggest ethnic group in Britain, which is white British (ONS, 2013). Difference manifests itself within healthcare as inequality experienced by 'other' groups and the detrimental effects this has on their lives. The government has acknowledged these 'other' groups and the inequality that they experience not only within healthcare, but within society as a whole. The Equality Act 2010 brought together previous legislation, such as the Equal Pay Act 1970 and the Employment Equality (Age) Regulations 2006, under one Act of Parliament (HM Government, 2013). The Act identified the following protected characteristics: age, disability, gender reassignment, race, religion or belief (including lack of belief), sex, and sexual orientation. These groups will be discussed throughout the book. It is interesting to note that this legislation uses the terms 'sex' and 'race', not 'gender' and 'ethnicity'. This creates even more blurred lines of meaning. This is something that, as nurses/midwives, you will have to grapple with on a daily basis as your patients' identities are wrapped up in these socially constructed categories.

Prejudice and stereotyping

In defining these two terms together, it is important to appreciate that they are inextricably linked to inequality in society, and therefore healthcare and healthcare systems. These are complex terms that have theoretically changed over time. Nelson (2009, 2015), a social psychologist, identifies prejudice as the negative attitude towards a group or towards a member of that group, and stereotyping as the traits that come to mind when we think of a group or an individual from that group that is different from another group. These differences can be based on ethnicity, religion, sexual orientation, and physical or mental abilities. There does not need to be an unequal power relationship for prejudice and stereotyping to be used by any group (Dovidio et al., 2010). However, they are inextricably linked to racism and racial discrimination, Islamophobia, anti-Semitism, homophobia and transphobia. This is where the importance of power plays an integral part in how the negative traits attributed to the formation of stereotypes of particular groups leads to prejudice and then racism (or Islamophobia or anti-Semitism). If one group, white, historically has more power based on slavery and colonisation over 'other' groups (e.g. BAME people), then the social construct of race leading to racism becomes a part of how people interact with each other in society. This includes healthcare, because people from society work and practise in healthcare. You bring these social constructs with you.

Racism and racial discrimination

There are many theories of racism that address the concept from a historical, sociological, political, legal and cultural perspective (Goldberg, 2015). Fredrickson (2015, pp19–28) picks up one of the main themes highlighted in this book, which is difference.

Within healthcare, the issue of difference is not only racially based, but also biased towards other socially disadvantaged groups, such as patients with learning disabilities or mental health problems. They become the 'them' to the 'normal' us. This allows us, as healthcare professionals, to treat 'different' patients from these groups in a way in which we would not treat others and ourselves.

Racial discrimination is often used interchangeably with racism. Solomos (2003) conceptualises that racial discrimination has three components: acts, processes and practice. There is someone responsible for acting in a racially discriminative manner and there are processes that are 'established, routine and subtle' (p77) within healthcare services. These acts of racial discrimination can be perpetrated by healthcare professionals and do have a significant impact on patient care, well-being and outcomes.

Difference, diversity and inequality in health

Diversity is a poly-functional term used to describe and analyze the complex dynamics in today's society.

(Braedel-Kühner and Müller, 2015, p7)

Professor Lorraine Culley of De Montfort University has written extensively on diverse groups' interactions and inequality within healthcare:

While these are highly disparate groups (and internally very heterogeneous), they share at least one important feature which each contribution ably demonstrates: their health is intimately bound up with the multi-faceted disadvantage that derives from the social, political and economic make-up of our society and our response to 'difference'.

(Culley, 2010, p299)

There are three issues here. Diverse groups have similarities, but this does not mean that each member of the group is the same and should be treated as individuals. These individuals and groups do not exist in a vacuum outside of societal external influences, such as class and income. As healthcare professionals, we must constantly challenge the idea that 'difference' can be reduced to people being simply unequal to the rest of 'normal' society. An acknowledgement of the complexities of diversity and difference is important in allowing nurses to treat the patient, not the difference as to which society labels people.

Activity 1.1 asks you to consider how ethnic diversity might affect you as a healthcare professional, and how this might affect how you interact and organise your care for a patient.

Activity 1.1 Reflection

Think about an occasion in the clinical environment that you have witnessed which you or the patient/service user has considered to be related to ethnicity in a negative way. How did it affect the care that you or your colleagues provided?

Why do you think it is important to be aware of these issues?

Although this activity is based on your own reflection, there is also a model answer provided at the end of the chapter.

Having considered how an awareness of the negative issues surrounding ethnic diversity might inform your practice, we now turn to *equity* and *equality*.

Equity and equality: are they the same?

There is a frequent misunderstanding that equity and equality are the same, and they are regularly used interchangeably, particularly when discussing health. The NHS principles are based both on equity and equality. Access to healthcare at the point of use regardless of ability to pay is the cornerstone of the NHS (National Health Service Act 1946). Equity is accepting that equal access does not mean equitable outcome as many diverse groups have unequitable access, treatment and outcomes that are in part or wholly based on diversity, and the marginalisation and discrimination that comes with it. For example, the LGBT community has experiences of marginalisation (Culley, 2010), and in general hospitals patients with learning disabilities have been discriminated against, which has led to death (Culley, 2010; Heslop et al., 2013; Mencap, 2013). Racial discrimination of BAME patients has led to poorer outcomes and experience of healthcare (EHRC, 2016b; Heslop et al., 2013). The key is that in society and health, all people do not start from the same position, and if diverse groups 'lag behind' from the beginning then more time or resources are needed to assure equity. When delivering care, this is something that you should consider. It is so important that the World Health Organization states:

Health inequities are avoidable inequalities in health between groups of people within countries and between countries. These inequities arise from inequalities within and between societies.

(WHO, 2008c, p1)

Once an acknowledgement of inequity in health has been established, we must then look at the possible reasons for this and the terminology that is used to describe it, both globally and here at home in the UK. The World Health Organization (WHO, 2008c) and the Marmot Review (Marmot et al., 2010) consider the following as important:

What are the social 'determinants' of health?

The social determinants of health are the circumstances in which people are born, grow up, live, work and age, and the systems put in place to deal with illness. These circumstances are in turn shaped by a wider set of forces: economics, social policies, and politics.

(WHO, 2008c)

What are the drivers of health inequalities?

The global context affects how societies prosper through its impact on international relations and domestic norms and policies. These in turn shape the way that society, both at the national and local level, organises its affairs, giving rise to forms of social position and hierarchy, whereby populations are organised according to income, education, occupation, gender, race/ethnicity and other factors. Where people are in the social hierarchy affects the conditions in which they grow, learn, live, work and age, their vulnerability to ill health, and the consequences of ill health.

(WHO, 2008c)

Marmot Review: Fair Society, Healthy Lives

Focusing solely on the most disadvantaged will not reduce health inequalities sufficiently. To reduce the steepness of the social gradient in health, actions must be universal, but with a scale and intensity that is proportionate to the level of disadvantage. We call this proportionate universalism.

Action taken to reduce health inequalities will benefit society in many ways. It will have economic benefits in reducing losses from illness associated with health inequalities. These currently account for productivity losses, reduced tax revenue, higher welfare payments and increased treatment costs.

In turn, these factors are influenced by social position, itself shaped by education, occupation, income, gender, ethnicity and race. All these influences are affected by the sociopolitical and cultural and social context in which they sit.

(Marmot et al., 2010)

The WHO and the Marmot Review have been highlighted among an ongoing and growing body of evidence on the issue of social determinants. Note the similarities between these reports. It is because of this similarity internationally and nationally that they have been used. The social determinants of health are linked to diverse groups. There is also a clear relationship between the social position of our patients and how this must be considered when managing patient care in conjunction with the patient.

Activity 1.2 specifically identifies that health inequalities exist for certain ethnic groups in British society, and what, if anything, can and should be done to redress this.

Activity 1.2 Evidence-based practice and research

Locate the National Institute for Health and Care Excellence's (NICE) guidance for preventing ill health and premature death in BAME groups: **www.nice.org.uk/guidance/ph46/chapter/3-Considerations**

Read through the web page and consider whether you knew that there was a difference in increased risk of diabetes due to body mass index (BMI) and that ethnicity makes such a difference. Evidence-based practice can make a clear link to differing ethnic groups having a higher risk of contracting a long-term condition such as diabetes. Therefore, if you are practising in an area with a high BAME population, information such as this must be something that you seek out. Ensure that you have the right information for the population in which you practise.

An outline of what you need to consider is given at the end of the chapter.

Diversity: statistical data and research findings

There is much statistical data on the diversity of the UK population, policy findings, and research on diversity and health. The following are significant and provide context to the patients you will encounter in practice:

- The population of the UK in mid-2018 was estimated to be 66,436,000 (ONS, 2019b).
- In the 2011 census, 58,000 people identified themselves as gypsy or Irish traveller (0.1 per cent of the usual resident population of England and Wales) (ONS, 2014).
- There are 12.9 million disabled people in the UK: 7 per cent of children, 17 per cent of working-age adults and 45 per cent of pension-age adults.
- In the 2011 census, the number of residents who stated that their religion was Christian in England and Wales was fewer than in 2001. The size of this group decreased by 12.4 per cent to 59.3 per cent (33.2 million) in 2011 from 71.7 per cent (37.3 million) in 2001 (ONS, 2012).
- In 2017, there were an estimated 1.1 million people aged 16 years and over identifying as LGB out of a UK population aged 16 years and over of 52.8 million. People aged 16 to 24 years were most likely to identify as LGB in 2017 (4.2 per cent). Males (2.3 per cent) were more likely to identify as LGB than females (1.8 per cent) in 2017 (ONS, 2019c).
- It is estimated that in England in 2015 there were 1,087,100 people with learning disabilities, including 930,400 adults (PHE, 2016).

The Equality and Human Rights Commission (EHRC, 2016a) has found the following:

- Among lesbian and bisexual women, 50 per cent of them have had negative experiences of the NHS.
- People with mental health problems have much higher rates of physical illness, with a range of factors contributing to greater prevalence of, and premature mortality from, coronary heart disease, stroke, diabetes, infections and respiratory disease.
- People with severe mental illness die, on average, 20 years younger than the general population, often from preventable physical illnesses.
- While the UK's white population has remained roughly the same size over the past ten years, the ethnic minority population has almost doubled, and now is at least 8 million people, or 14 per cent of the UK population.
- The proportion of UK citizens from ethnic minority communities is expected to double in the next decades and will be between 20 and 30 per cent by 2050.

Furthermore:

- Compared with the general population, gypsies and travellers are more likely to suffer bad health. This includes lower life expectancy, high infant mortality rates, high maternal mortality rates, low child immunisation levels, higher prevalence of anxiety and depression, chronic cough or bronchitis (even after smoking is taken into account), asthma, chest pain and diabetes (DCLG, 2012), and higher rates of smoking (Aspinall, 2014). This is exacerbated by the fact that many gypsies and travellers remain unregistered with GPs (RCGP, 2013).
- People with learning disabilities die, on average, 15–20 years sooner than people in the general population, with some of these deaths identified as being potentially amenable to good-quality healthcare (University of Bristol, 2018, p5).
- Mencap (2013) notes the following in relation to those with learning disabilities in acute hospitals:

Our cases show that, despite some encouraging evidence of a better understanding of the concept of reasonable adjustments across the NHS, a lack of compliance with the Disability Discrimination Act (now the Equality Act) underpins the failures identified by families. They illustrate both direct discrimination from NHS staff and a failure to take the steps required by the law. These failings, combined with a striking lack of compliance with the Mental Capacity Act, make it clear that the very people this legislation was designed to protect remain at risk.

(p8)

Intersectionality: health and diversity

Crenshaw's (1989) original use of the term intersectionality was to explain the intersecting effects of race and gender on black women in legal cases, and that the effects of being both female and black worked together to cause disadvantage in the American legal system. Here, the focus is not only on being female and black, but other social categories of marginalised groups who experience health inequalities: the LGBTQ community, people with learning disabilities and mental health issues, and religions that have a history of being marginalised in Western Christian society, such as Judaism and Islam. Intersectionality can be used as an analytical tool to understand the wider context of the human experience in society (Collins and Bilge, 2016) and in healthcare (Green et al., 2017).

Case study: An Asian woman with learning disabilities

Jatinder Kaur is a 25-year-old British Asian Sikh woman with a mild learning disability who lives at home with her parents. She has a good support network of her parents, family and friends, a full social life, and a part-time job. She is admitted to a surgical ward with moderate to severe lower abdominal pain, nausea and vomiting. Jatinder's pain is not being controlled effectively; she is crying out periodically in an unusual way, and her family are worried and concerned as they have never seen her behave like this when unwell and have informed the nurse that this indicates something seriously wrong. Mathew is the registered nurse working in the bay of patients in which Jatinder is located. He is finding it difficult to manage all the relatives and it is hard to interpret her behaviour in relation to pain, especially with intravenous morphine having been given for the pain 30 minutes ago. He has nursed 'Asian patients' before and a few patients that have learning disabilities, and Jatinder is not acting in the way he is expecting.

The intersecting issues here are ethnicity, culture, religion, learning disabilities and gender. Together they can make the 'perfect storm' of discrimination, leading to poor care delivery and outcome for Jatinder's care. Non-white patients and those with learning disabilities have poorer health outcomes (Emerson et al., 2016; Robertson et al., 2015) based on racial and unconscious bias, prejudice, and discrimination by health professionals (Dovidio and Fiske, 2012; Drewniak et al., 2017; FitzGerald and Hurst, 2017). Jatinder's ability to convey her needs to healthcare professionals based on her learning disability and family members or carers not being listened to means that assessment of care around pain management can be poor, which increases her risk of deteriorating without the appropriate interventions. Women's account of presenting symptoms, particularly BAME women, has been problematised by the assessment and planning of care not being appropriate for their needs (Andrews et al., 2017).

Research summary: unconscious bias in healthcare

The goal for healthcare professionals is to consistently deliver safe, competent care equitably to all patients (NMC, 2015). Individualised patient-centred care delivery is the cornerstone of modern healthcare (McCormack and McCance, 2016). Unconscious bias, or implicit bias as it can also be called, is a significant barrier to achieving this (Holm et al., 2017). We all have biases and stereotypes about people and groups that can be based on culture (Schultz and Baker, 2017), race and ethnicity (Holm et al., 2017), and physical and mental impairment. Bucknor-Ferron and Zagaja (2016) define unconscious bias as 'the multifaceted evaluation of one group and its members relative to another' (p61). The evaluation is unconscious; you are not directly aware that you are delivering care inadequately because of negative stereotyping based on preconceived ideas and expectations of an individual or group's behaviour. Care is poor because unconscious bias affects clinical decision-making and interactions between patient and healthcare professional, and within the systems and processes of a health organisation and its staff (FitzGerald and Hurst, 2017; Kapur, 2015).

Activity 1.3 looks at a clinical encounter where unconscious bias could impact negatively on decision-making.

Activity 1.3   Reflection

Think about how you expect a person to behave in certain circumstances:

* when they are a patient in pain;
* when they are a grieving relative; and
* when they are a patient being taught how to take their blood glucose level.

Now think about how ethnicity, sexuality or religion added to any of these situations might change how you behave in each of these cases without you even thinking that they do. If that behaviour discriminates against that patient or family members in a negative way, that behaviour could be attributed to unconscious bias. This in turn can have a bad effect on the patient's experience, healthcare delivery and health outcome.

An outline of what you might find is given at the end of the chapter.

Bucknor-Ferron and Zagaja (2016) ask healthcare professionals to consider the following points in order to reduce unconscious bias:

* *Personal awareness and acknowledgement*: an ability to look at yourself and be aware that you hold these biases.
* *Empathy*: an ability to understand what your patients are feeling and experiencing.

- *Advocacy*: supporting your patients as they move through the health service.
- *Education*: learning formally on your course and learning from others and yourself from your own experiences.

These are attributes that, as a student, you should be fine-tuning, and will continue to do so throughout your career.

Let us now look at what you have gained from this chapter.

Chapter summary

This chapter has considered the concept of diversity, what it means in terms of various social groups within the UK, and how its meaning has changed. The chapter has introduced important terms, such as 'race', 'culture', 'ethnicity' and 'unconscious bias'. The vital importance of social determinants of health has been discussed, showing how they can lead to poor health outcomes for patients from diverse backgrounds. Finally, the chapter introduced the term 'intersectionality' as a means of linking together different aspects of people's identity. We saw how, without an understanding of intersectionality, it can increase the risk of poor clinical decision-making and lead to inequity and inequality of care.

Activities: brief outline answers

Activity 1.1   Reflection (p12)

Think of how ethnic diversity could affect care delivery.

Racial discrimination, Islamophobia and unconscious bias can lead healthcare professionals to make poor clinical decisions due to how you or colleagues may behave towards these groups detrimentally, making poor clinical decisions or restricting access to services.

An example of what you might have witnessed could be the treatment of a young African Caribbean man with mental health problems seen as more threatening and violent than his white male counterpart in an emergency department, a ward or in the patient's home.

It is important to have sufficient knowledge of how some ethnic groups are more susceptible to specific health-related issues (e.g. genetic conditions such as sickle-cell anaemia in people of African and Caribbean descent, and an increased risk of prostate cancer in African Caribbean men – one in four – compared to white men – one in eight).

Activity 1.2   Evidence-based practice and research (p14)

The guidance uses evidence to support that the BMI of BAME people should be used differently than the white population, as BAME groups suffer from adverse health outcomes in relation to diabetes at a lower BMI than the white population in the UK. If you are working in an area that has a high BAME population, it is in the best interests of your patients that you are familiar with this type of evidence-based information with which to make an appropriate decision and offer health advice.

Activity 1.3   Reflection (p17)

There are differences in how cultural and ethnic groups as well as genders express pain and are assessed for pain. If your expectation is not attuned to this, you may not assess pain levels appropriately, and this could have serious patient care implication.

You might react inappropriately to differing expressions of grief by a bereaved person, which can worsen the experience of the death of a loved one.

You might have an expectation that certain ethnic groups or patients with learning disabilities are going to be more 'hard work' or 'difficult to teach' than white middle-class patients who do not have a learning disability. The spectrum of learning disabilities must be understood before assuming that a patient with a learning disability cannot be taught certain skills.

Further reading

Bucknor-Ferron, P. and Zagaja, L. (2016) Five strategies to combat unconscious bias. *Nursing,* 46(11): 61–2.

This article is an excellent piece on unconscious bias in healthcare. The writers identify groups that unconscious bias affects and the different types of bias that exist, as well as how unconscious bias affects clinical decisions and what as health professionals we can try to do to eliminate it from our decision-making.

Garner, S. (2017) *Racism: An Introduction* (2nd edn). London: SAGE.

This book is a recent publication and a sound introduction to discussions and theories of race. It is not healthcare-specific, but this does give you more insight into some of the areas we have mentioned or discussed, such as ethnicity, race and Islamophobia.

Scriven, A. (2017) *Ewles & Simnett's Promoting Health: A Practical Guide* (7th edn). Oxford: Elsevier Health.

This is a well-established book in the field of health promotion, and Chapter 2 has some important points to make on the inequalities of health in an accessible and informative way.

Useful websites

The Marmot Review: Fair Society Healthy Lives

www.instituteofhealthequity.org/resources-reports/fair-society-healthy-lives-the-marmot-review

This is an important report that deserves further reading as contemporary discussions of health inequality internationally and here in the UK cannot be understood without being familiar with this groundbreaking report. Professor Sir Michael Marmot is highly respected in the field of inequality and health and has researched and written extensively on this topic.

Mencap

www.mencap.org.uk/learning-disability-explained/what-learning-disability

This is the website for the charity whose main objective is to support people and their families with learning disabilities (LDs). This page looks at some issues discussed in this chapter. It is useful for healthcare professionals and the public alike. It has information on projects run for people with LDs to research and statistics on how to improve the lives and care required for people with LDs.

Office for National Statistics (ONS)

www.ons.gov.uk

The ONS is the UK's largest independent producer of official statistics and the recognised national statistical institute of the UK. It is the organisation that collates the data from the population census that are collected every ten years. For a breakdown of the population by ethnic origin, if born in the UK or outside the UK, age range of the population, gender breakdown, and issues related to health, this is the place to go.

World Health Organization (WHO)

www.who.int

The WHO began when its constitution came into force on 7 April 1948, and works with its 194 member states, across six regions, from more than 150 offices. WHO staff are united in a shared commitment to achieve better health for everyone, everywhere. They strive to combat diseases – communicable diseases such as influenza and HIV, and non-communicable diseases such as cancer and heart disease. For ideas of how UK health concerns relate to international health, this is an invaluable resource.

Chapter 2 Diversity and cultural concepts of health

Beverley Brathwaite

NMC Standards of Proficiency for Registered Nurses

This chapter will address the following platforms and proficiencies:

Platform 1: Being an accountable professional

1.9 understand the need to base all decisions regarding care and interventions on people's needs and preferences, recognising and addressing any personal and external factors that may unduly influence their decisions.

Platform 2: Promoting health and preventing ill health

2.2 demonstrate knowledge of epidemiology, demography, genomics and the wider determinants of health, illness and wellbeing and apply this to an understanding of global patterns of health and wellbeing outcomes.

Platform 7: Coordinating care

7.9 facilitate equitable access to healthcare for people who are vulnerable or have a disability, demonstrate the ability to advocate on their behalf when required, and make necessary reasonable adjustments to the assessment, planning and delivery of their care.

Chapter aims

After reading this chapter, you will be able to:

- explain what health is and how it relates to diverse members of the population;
- define the terms 'epidemiology', 'demography' and 'genomics';
- understand how stigma relates to healthcare outcomes for diverse groups; and
- understand determinants of health and inequality of health, and the impact of these within diverse groups.

Introduction

> ## Case study: Cunningham Street
>
> Let us go back to Cunningham Street, with its inhabitants of differing ethnicities, cultures, faiths, religions, sexualities and intellectual abilities. At no. 35 lives Anish, of Asian descent, and his wife is due her first annual smear test. Karen at no. 12 has been experiencing vaginal discharge for the past month and is worried, but she is reluctant to go to the GP as the practice nurse was previously asking unrelated questions about her personal life with her wife. At the GP practice at the end of the street, a middle-aged man who identifies himself as Roma is trying to get an appointment with the GP due to ongoing pain in his joints. At no. 2, Olufunke's mother, who is of Nigerian descent, has high blood pressure. At no. 5, Jennifer, who is a young woman of Caribbean descent and is on the autistic spectrum, is worried about her friend Olufemi who has sickle-cell anaemia.
>
> The residents on Cunningham Street all have health needs that require evidence-based clinical knowledge that is specific to their ethnicity, culture, sexuality and intellectual abilities.

In Chapter 2, we will be addressing health as a concept and how this has changed over time, as well as the experiences of health and healthcare of differing members of the community. The relationships that the residents of Cunningham Street have within society, and how these connect to healthcare delivery, life expectancy, health outcomes and negative experiences that can occur from healthcare professionals, as well as the drivers for these experiences, will be examined. We will also consider health both internationally and nationally from a diversity perspective. People and communities such as the LGBTQ community, adults with learning disabilities, and ethnic groups such as gypsy Roma travellers and those of African Caribbean and South Asian descent are more susceptible to certain health conditions, outcomes, experiences of healthcare and differing life expectancy than the general population. These will be discussed further. Reasons for inequitable experiences, such as determinants of health, stigmatisation, and stereotyping based on ethnicity, gender and class, will be examined. The legislation used to combat discrimination and the terminology used will be addressed.

What is health?

Health is considered to be one of our most important values. Many people in modern times regard health as one of the most precious values in life (Nordenfelt, 2007). However, for some diverse groups, health is experienced in differing ways. It is important to understand how stigma, determinants of health, and social determinants work together to influence the health outcomes and personal experiences of diverse patients. It is influenced by international evidence and guidance, government and local policy, and individual interactions. It may seem that you have little control over all of this, but you have more influence than you think. You represent the NHS every day and your interaction with patients makes a significant difference. This should never be underestimated. The more positive the interactions are between your patients and their family, significant others, or carers can make an enormous difference to their health in the short and long term. Therefore, this chapter will endeavour to bring together international ideas and key terms that heavily influence legislation, policy and care delivery that affect all patients and service users. It will take into consideration the distinctive needs of certain diverse groups. First, let us look at the idea of what 'health' means and how this has changed over time by considering definitions from a variety of organisations:

A state of complete physical, mental, and social well-being, and not merely the absence of disease and infirmity.

(WHO, 1948)

Health is not just about the presence of disease or illness (be that physical or mental), but also about how well people are. Nor is health just about individuals. Taking a population view is important for understanding potential threats to our health.

(Department of Health, 2010b, p5)

Health is a dynamic state of wellbeing that occurs, when biologically given and personally acquired potentials together fulfil the demands of life.

(Sturmberg, 2014, p415)

The breaking down of the components of health into the physical (biological composition), social (social roles/interactions and spiritual) and mental (psychological, emotional, and mental status of the individual) health.

(Alslman et al., 2015)

A healthy person is someone with the opportunity for meaningful work, secure housing, stable relationships, high self-esteem and healthy behaviours. A healthy society, in turn, is not one that waits for people to become ill, but one that sees how health is shaped by social, cultural, political, economic, commercial and environmental factors, and acts on these for current and future generations.

(Health Foundation, 2018, p7)

There has been a shift away from the term 'complete' used by the World Health Organization (WHO, 1948), which would indicate that if you have a manageable long-term condition you could be considered not to be healthy. There is a need to acknowledge that health is not static, and will need to incorporate cultural factors and the ability for people to re-establish a sense of well-being that may have shifted due to physical, mental and social changes (Huber et al., 2011). The transformation of what health can mean has coincided with the change in the diversity of the population both internationally and here in the UK. In parts of the country, differing ethnic, cultural and religious groups interact with each other as never before. The Health Foundation (2018) gives a broader idea of health within the context of the patient being a member of society, focusing on how that person interacts in society, and considers what can be done to reduce ill health before it happens, with a clear acknowledgement of how society can shape how this happens.

The study of demography is the study of human populations with respect to their size, structure and dynamics. For demographers, a population is a group of individuals that coexist at a point in time and share a defining characteristic, such as residence in the same geographical area. The structure or composition of a population refers to the distribution of its members by age, sex, ethnicity and other characteristics, such as being lesbian, gay, bisexual, transgender and queer (LGBTQ) or having a learning disability (LD). Demography and health can give us a better understanding of the distribution of health within a given region and group. With this information, decisions about how, where and on whom resources are spent can be made. We will take some time to look at health issues related to these groups.

Gypsy Roma travellers

Gypsy Roma travellers (GRTs) are now part of the census data; they were finally added as an ethnic group in the 2011 census, making up 0.1 per cent (58,000) of the population (ONS, 2014), although it is possible the number is higher, up to 200,000 (Gill et al., 2013). There has been continued research taking place into their healthcare needs (Burchardt et al., 2018), the most important aspect of which is accommodation – access to safe and clean sites for caravans (Aspinall, 2014).

There are multiple issues related to health and social exclusion that are experienced by GRTs. They are more prone to long-term conditions, a higher perinatal infant mortality rate of all ethnic minority populations, higher levels of stress, anxiety, depression and smoking, and increased alcohol consumption (Cromarty, 2018; Gill et al., 2013). They suffer poorer physical health and poorer access to health and primary care services (EHRC, 2016a). For the GRT community, accessing healthcare is difficult. One reason is their nomadic lifestyle, which means that registering with a GP, and even access to a dentist, can be a challenge. The health issues for this community run throughout the life course from birth, with this group having the highest maternal death rate of any ethnic group, and young children are more at risk due to lower immunisation rates. Not all GRTs live in caravans, but when they do live in houses it can be in areas of higher deprivation, and health outcomes do not necessarily improve (Aspinall, 2014; Gill et al., 2013). Greenfields (2017, p25) identified practical and administrative challenges for GRTs, as well as a lack of appropriate documentation, including adequate citizenship documentation, which affects entitlement to services following recent migration and entitlement to welfare. Limited access to or awareness of NHS entitlement is exacerbated by low literacy levels. It is also worth adding that evidence suggests racial discrimination 'exacerbates the inequalities they continually experience' (Cromarty, 2018, p23).

Lesbian, gay, bisexual, transgender and queer

Globally, the LGBTQ community must combat violence and criminalisation (Lo and Horton, 2016), same-sex relationships are illegal in 72 countries, and in eight countries just being homosexual is punishable by death (Duncan, 2017). Although transgender people have existed across history and cultures throughout the world, transgenderism and transsexualism are considered abnormal in many societies as they diverge from the normative male–female binary that exists predominantly across the world (Wylie et al., 2016). The United Nations High Commissioner for Human Rights states that human rights law is obligated to protect all people from discrimination on the grounds of gender identity. This is not always the case, and to determine the experiences of the LGBTQ community in the UK, the Government Equalities Office carried out a national survey in 2018.

In relation to Platform 7.13 of the NMC code, it is necessary for you, as a student, to appreciate the political context and wider determinants of health from which your patients come and in which they find themselves with you and the NHS. For example, the fear of physical violence is an unacceptable reality for many in the LGBTQ community in Europe and the UK (Clark, 2014). The damaging effects of hate crimes against members of the LGBTQ community not only affect their physical, but also their emotional and psychological, well-being (Jurcic, 2016). Therefore, your first encounter with an LGBTQ patient could be in the emergency department, where physical needs would need to be addressed, but this could also be an opportunity to help with emotional and psychological needs. Overall, heterosexuals fare better in healthcare, while bisexuals have the worst experiences, and gay and lesbian people have poorer mental health (Booker et al., 2017). In the longer term, it may be that mental health services are best suited to support the emotional and psychological trauma that can result from experiences of being part of the LGBTQ community. For example, there is a higher risk of suicide and attempted suicide (Peate, 2016). This must not be underestimated as a significant and possible outcome if appropriate support and interventions are not put in place. Bachmann and Gooch (2019), the RCN (2016a) and Robinson (2019) have acknowledged the discrimination that LGBTQ patients experience from healthcare professionals. The RCN (2016a) has provided a clear policy to reduce this discrimination. It is your responsibility and accountability once registered with the NMC to deliver care equitably. Bristowe et al. (2018) found that the impact of discrimination on the LGBTQ community's health covers their life span. They have a higher risk of some cancers and greater all-cause mortality than heterosexual people. They often present later in the treatment and disease pathway, have unmet bereavement needs, and have a higher rate of mental illness and risky behaviours (e.g. drinking, smoking, drug use) that are linked to discrimination. This discrimination could lead to a reluctance in adhering to effective follow-up or community care and experiencing poor levels of care while in treatment (Glasper, 2016; RCN, 2016a).

Learning disabilities

Current knowledge indicates that the reasons for the poorer health of people with intellectual disabilities primarily fall within two broad spheres. First, a range of secondary health conditions is associated with some specific causes of intellectual disabilities. Second, people with intellectual disability are much more likely than their non-disabled peers to be exposed to a range of well-established social determinants of poorer health (e.g. poverty, social exclusion, discrimination, reduced access to timely and effective healthcare) (Emerson et al., 2014, p592). These are the stark and unacceptable realities of children and adults with learning disabilities. British adults with learning disabilities have a distinctly poorer quality of health than their non-disabled peers (Emerson et al., 2012, 2016; Hatton et al., 2017; HQIP, 2017). There is also a higher relationship between physical and mental health problems within those with learning disabilities than the general population (Hatton et al., 2017). As a student nurse of any field, adult, child, mental health, and of course LD, it is extremely likely that you will be providing care for a patient with an LD, and in a variety of differing healthcare settings within a hospital environment, surgery and emergency department. The community setting is also an area for care delivery for many patients with learning disabilities in their home and specialised care facilities. The multidisciplinary team (MDT) is, not surprisingly, frequently utilised in care delivery with patients who have mild to severe learning disabilities.

As a member of the MDT, it is important that you know who the other members are and what their role is in delivering care holistically to the patient, carers and family. You will need to know when to refer and the reason for the referral. Activity 2.1 will allow you to think about which members of the MDT are involved.

Activity 2.1 Team-working

Make a list of the MDT members who can be involved in the care of patients with learning disabilities and what role they would take in their care.

An outline of what you might find is given at the end of the chapter.

Activity 2.1 demonstrates that you must have identified multiple members of the MDT with whom you have worked already or know of the vital role they play. The need to work as a member of the healthcare team in providing the best possible care for this group of patients is an ongoing skill, as new roles are developed particularly to enhance care for patients with learning disabilities.

Due to medical and societal advancement, there has been an increase in the life expectancy of people with learning disabilities (PHE, 2016; Welsh Government, 2018). This has its benefits, but it has increased the risk of certain long-term conditions and physical conditions that are associated with learning disabilities. For example, congenital heart failure affects nearly 50 per cent of all people with Down syndrome, autism and psychiatric disorder have a strong link, and respiratory disease is the leading cause of death (Emerson and Baines, 2011). Being aware of the key health problems associated within the learning disability community is imperative when assessing their nursing needs as accurately as possible. Emerson and Baines (2011) have identified the specific areas shown in Table 2.1.

Respiratory disease
Coronary heart disease
Cancer
Mental health and challenging behaviour
Dementia
Epilepsy
Sensory impairment
Physical impairment
Oral health
Dysphagia
Constipation
Osteoporosis
Endocrine disorders
Diabetes
Injury, accidents and falls
Gastro-oesophageal reflux disease

Table 2.1   Health problems associated with learning disability

Due to these complex issues, many people with learning disabilities can have more difficulties identifying health problems and getting treatment for them. As a response, annual learning disability health checks have been a key part of NHS plans to improve health and reduce premature mortality since 2008 (Hatton et al., 2017). Communication, as well as patients not understanding what is happening to them and why, can make it difficult for you to make an accurate clinical decision. With learning disabilities, there is not always a physical attribute that may indicate that a learning disability affects your patient. Even if there is such an attribute, it can be challenging to ascertain their level of understanding of what they are being told or asked. This could easily be misunderstood as incomprehension or uncooperativeness. Hatton et al. (2017) state that 'there may be uncertainty over patients' capacity to consent to interventions and a lack of understanding of the legal requirements for proxy decision making if they cannot' (p24). The involvement of the patient, family, carer, and/or social or key worker is vital to ensure safe care delivery.

Diversity: epidemiology, demography and genomics

There are key terms within Platform 2.2 that deserve to be addressed as they can be aligned to the understanding of issues relating to the changing British population. Demography is the way in which a population is studied to determine the causes of health and disease. Key components of studying the demography of a population are morbidity, mortality, migration, ethnicity, class and gender. Epidemiology has a close relationship to demography as it is the study of a population and how often disease occurs in differing groups within that population. An example would be to consider a single group, women or men, and then look even closer by separating out women by ethnic group or age and determining what disease or illness rates occur in these particular groups, and what targeted prevention or care delivery needs to be arranged. Women over 50 years old should go for breast screening every three years as the risk of breast cancer increases (NHS, 2019). Some black, Asian and minority ethnic (BAME) women are less likely to take up this screening compared to their white counterparts, indicating a need to target campaigns at specific ethnic groups (Vrinten et al., 2016). This is an example of the importance of demographic and epidemiological knowledge in targeting healthcare delivery for diverse groups.

Genomics incorporates and identifies that multiple genes work together with environmental influences, resulting in a situation of health or illness. Nurses will increasingly be called upon to use genetic- and genomic-based approaches and technologies in client care (Lea, 2009, p1). However, even here there is inequality, as only 2 per cent of the Human Genome Project has been collected from Africa, meaning less opportunities to use genomics to aid specific and effective treatments for Africans and patients of African descent (Mabuka-Maroa, 2019).

Activity 2.2 Evidence-based practice and research

Go to the Genomics Education Programme web page on the Health Education England website: **www.genomicseducation.hee.nhs.uk/resources/genetic-conditions-factsheets/**

Look for the following genetic conditions: sickle-cell anaemia, alpha thalassemia.

Find out:

1. What ethnic groups are more likely to have the condition?
2. What is given as the reason for the genetic condition?
3. What is the clinical management of the condition?

An outline of what you might find is given at the end of the chapter.

Some genetic-based conditions have a strong connection to ethnic and cultural groups. Activity 2.2 will get you to look at sickle-cell anaemia and find out more about this genetic condition and the ethnic groups in which it is more likely to be found.

As you can see from Activity 2.2, Health Education England is a resource not only for healthcare professionals, but patients and family members, and it can be used as an additional source of information. Accessing varied forms of health information in differing formats improves health literacy, particularly for diverse groups. This is looked at in more detail in Chapter 7.

The ethnic demography of an area will increase the possibility of certain genetic conditions being prevalent, and in turn the need for the use of local primary and secondary services. As a nurse working in certain parts of the country, it is in your and your patients' best interests that you are familiar with these genetic conditions to ensure that competent care can be given. These are conditions that will require lifelong support and medical and nursing interventions not only for the physical symptoms, but the psychological symptoms that can coexist with them, such as depression (Jonassaint et al., 2016; Wallen et al., 2014). There is also a cultural context. For example, patients with sickle-cell anaemia can have negative experiences in hospital services and care delivery (Haywood et al., 2014). These patients and their family members can feel shame, blame themselves or see sickle-cell anaemia as a curse (Burnes et al., 2008). As a nurse, it is your responsibility to respond to these ideas in a respectful manner but to support patients in moving away from these negative feelings. Giving clear information on the genetic reasons for sickle-cell anaemia, as well as referring to the appropriate specialist nurse in hospital and out in the community to ensure continued support, is of paramount importance to the ongoing well-being of patients with sickle-cell anaemia.

Stigma

There is a common thread running within the discussion in this chapter that affects diverse groups, and that is stigma. Stigma refers to the negative regard, inferior status and relative powerlessness that society collectively accords to people who possess a particular characteristic or belong to a particular group or category (Frost, 2011). Inherent in this definition is that stigma constitutes shared knowledge about which attributes and categories are valued by society and which ones are denigrated (Nelson, 2009). Stigma includes not only discrimination, but other 'parts', highlighted in Figure 2.1.

They work together and detrimentally influence treatment, access and experience (Richman and Hatzenbuehler, 2014). It is always people who stigmatise other people (Goldberg, 2017). This is no more evident than in healthcare. In Chapter 1, we looked at unconscious bias, prejudice, stereotyping and discrimination, and these 'parts' are linked to stigma, particularly in healthcare delivery, an overlapping that is clearly seen in Figure 2.1. In this chapter, we have looked at the LGBTQ, GRT, learning disability and

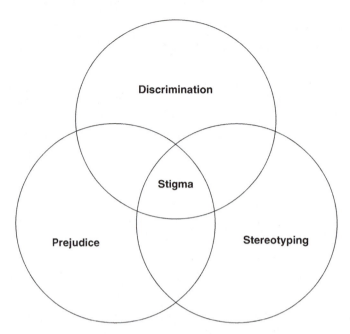

Figure 2.1 Stigmatisation – social constructs that work together in detrimentally influencing how healthcare professionals provide treatment

BAME communities. In one way or another, they all experience stigma or other significant social constructs, such as racism or those that are shown in Figure 2.1. The LGBTQ community faces discrimination and being stigmatised so much so that they fear informing health professionals of their sexuality because they have experienced homophobia (Clark, 2014; Fish and Evans, 2016), which in turn can harm health because people in this community are more likely to approach a health professional later in the progress of symptoms and illness (Richman and Hatzenbuehler, 2014). In the learning disability community, stigma not only harms care for the patient, but the family can also be stigmatised. Werner and Shulman (2015) call this 'stigma by association' (p272). As a result, the voiced concerns of the family and main carers for people with learning disabilities may be ignored, with disastrous consequences, which can and have led to the unnecessary death of patients with learning disabilities (University of Bristol, 2019). The gypsy and traveller population numbers in England and Wales are just under 60,000, but there are estimates that the numbers are as high as 200,000. Roma will only be added to the census data in 2021 (ONS, 2014; Parliament UK, 2019). The GRT community experiences racism, discrimination and being stigmatised at an unprecedented level. They experience social deprivation, low literacy and educational attainment (Cromarty, 2018). The NHS and healthcare professionals encounter significant challenges to meet the complex GRT healthcare needs caused by these experiences. Healthcare professionals can be judgemental, and their lack of cultural awareness is likely to be influenced by the media reinforcing stereotypes of poor behaviour and bad attributes of the GRT community (EHRC, 2016a; Gill et al., 2013). As with other minority groups, this can lead to them accessing health services later in the progression of their health problem, and consequently poorer outcomes from treatment.

As a student, you may already have witnessed this in the clinical setting in the varied interactions that take place on a daily basis between the nurse, patient, and significant others such as family carers and support workers. Without a clear understanding of how stigma and other social constructs inhibit a patient's treatment, any attempt at altering the way diverse individuals and groups are treated in the NHS will never change, and unacceptable clinical decisions will continue to be made.

As a student nurse, you must look at your own unconscious and implicit biases that can lead to stigmatisation of your patients. This is unacceptable practice that must be worked on constantly as you have a duty of care to your patients that is non-discriminatory. Stigma should have no place in your clinical decision-making process.

An example of a situation that can arise in the clinical environment can help to give you an idea of how stigma can influence communication and clinical decisions.

Scenario: Communication

You are a third-year adult nursing student on your final placement before finishing your degree. Olufemi is a 25-year-old British African man; he is well over six feet tall and well built, and it looks like he works out regularly. He is admitted overnight to your acute medical ward placement in sickle-cell crisis. He has not had a severe crisis that required admitting to hospital since his late teens, and this is his first time being admitted to an adult ward. On the morning shift with your practice supervisor in handover at 7.30 a.m., he is said to be in a little pain and is 'a bit needy like a lot of "sicklers" are'. He has intravenous morphine prescribed every two hours, which is just about managing his pain, and he has intravenous fluids running over eight hours. When you both go on to the ward after handover, Olufemi is in terrible pain, particularly in his legs, which have suddenly worsened. He is ringing the bell and calling out in pain when you enter the bay. Your practice supervisor goes straight to the call bell and turns it off, and tells him to try to be a little quieter as the noise he is making is disturbing the other patients. Before you and your practice supervisor have a chance to do anything else, Olufemi angrily states that you are more concerned about the noise he is making than the excruciating pain he is experiencing; he wants some painkillers now, and after this he wants to go home as he would be better off there than in here, where his illness is not understood and 'the care is rubbish'. Your practice supervisor replies to the patient that she is going to get the doctor to speak to him and does not engage in any other form of communication with Olufemi. She asks you to take his vital signs and walks away, saying to you, 'I don't have to take being spoken to like that by that type of patient'. You introduce yourself to him and ask if you can take his vital signs; he continues to be angry and says, 'Go the hell away and just get me my painkillers, I can't take this pain anymore'.

From this scenario, now turn to Activity 2.3.

Activity 2.3   Decision-making

From what was said in handover and by your practice supervisor considering issues of gender, ethnicity and Olufemi's sickle-cell disorder, what is being stigmatised?

Olufemi is obviously angry. Why do you think this is?

What could you and your practice supervisor do to improve this situation?

An outline of what you might answer is given at the end of the chapter.

In the above scenario and in Activity 2.3, we have looked at the possible experience of a black man of African descent in the NHS. Now we will look at the BAME community and how they view their health.

A portrait of modern Britain: the BAME experience

A report from Policy Exchange (Sunak and Rajeswaran, 2014) provides some valuable data on the BAME population in the UK, and the chapter on health is particularly useful. When self-reporting on their general health, most major ethnic groups had above-average proportions of people stating that they were in very good or good health. The black Caribbean community was a slightly negative outlier, and the black African community a slightly positive outlier. All ethnic minorities self-report good or very good levels of health, higher than the proportion of the white population (see Table 2.2).

	Very good or good	Fair	Bad or very bad
White	80%	14%	6%
Indian	85%	11%	4%
Pakistani	83%	11%	5%
Bangladeshi	83%	11%	6%
Black African	92%	6%	2%
Black Caribbean	77%	16%	7%

Table 2.2   Self-reported health status

Source: Sunak and Rajeswaran (2014, p56)

However, there are specific illnesses to which ethnic minorities are disproportionately susceptible, such as diabetes for South Asians and high blood pressure and stroke for black Africans and Caribbeans (see Table 2.3). Therefore, they are more likely to come into contact with you and the NHS than their white counterparts with these conditions, even when they state that their general health is good or very good.

	Asthma	Arthritis	Heart disease	Angina	Diabetes	High blood pressure	Depression
White	14%	16%	2.0%	3.3%	6%	20%	7%
Indian	9%	7%	1.3%	1.1%	9%	12%	2%
Pakistani	12%	7%	1.0%	3.0%	9%	9%	4%
Bangladeshi	10%	5%	1.9%	1.2%	10%	12%	2%
Black African	13%	11%	0.6%	1.0%	10%	21%	4%
Black Caribbean	6%	3%	0.1%	0.5%	3%	11%	2%

Table 2.3 Incidence of various health issues among different ethnic populations

Source: Sunak and Rajeswaran (2014, p58)

The reasons for these variables are multifaceted, and more research is required (Blom et al., 2016; Sunak and Rajeswaran, 2014). On a macro level, the richer the country is does not automatically translate to better health outcomes for BAME people, but a welfare state can make some improvements (Blom et al., 2016). What can we do, as nurses, to manage care for one of the statistically highest illnesses that affects the BAME community, diabetes? Research by Jhita et al. (2014) found that the quality of life for South Asians with diabetes is lower than their white participants. There is also a lack of understanding of the African Caribbean diet by healthcare professionals (Trueland, 2014). The need to understand the culture of your patients, and incorporating this into your care, is key to making care more equitable and patient-centred.

Determinants of health

Many different factors contribute to a person's current state of health. These factors may be biological, socio-economic, psychosocial, behavioural or social in nature. Scientists generally recognise five determinants of health of a population:

- *Biology and genetics. Examples: sex and age.*
- *Individual behavior. Examples: alcohol use, injection drug use (needles), unprotected sex, and smoking.*
- *Social environment. Examples: discrimination, income, and gender.*
- *Physical environment. Examples: where a person lives and crowded conditions.*
- *Health services. Examples: access to quality healthcare and having or not having health insurance.*

(Centers for Disease Control and Prevention, 2014)

These wider and individual issues must be taken into consideration as some of our patients will come from parts of the world where the health service and physical environment is considerably different than here in the UK. Also, in the UK, physical and social environments differ greatly. There are parts of the UK where the life expectancy is as low as poorer parts of the world. A highly cited example is what has been called the 'Glasgow effect'. In 2001, a boy in the deprived area of Calton in Glasgow had an average life expectancy of 54 years, compared with a boy from the affluent area of Lenzie, 12 km away in East Dunbartonshire, who could expect to live to 82 (WHO, 2011). However, things have changed, and the life expectancy of a male in Calton and Bridgeton shows that life expectancy has risen in recent years but has remained below the Glasgow average. In the period between 2008 and 2012, male life expectancy at birth was estimated by the Glasgow Centre for Population Health to be 67.8 years (Whyte, 2018), an obvious noteworthy increase. One factor that is likely to have contributed to the low life expectancy estimate at the time was that there were clusters of deaths in the area associated with the presence of particular hostels that looked after adults with a variety of problems related to drugs, alcohol, homelessness and mental health (Whyte, 2018).

Social determinants of health

The World Health Organization (WHO, 2008b) has made it its core business to address social determinants of health internationally. As can be observed, the social determinants of health are only one area covered by the determinants of health. The importance of these social determinants on diverse groups cannot be underestimated.

To give your local area of work some global context, it would be worthwhile looking at the Commission on Social Determinants of Health's final report: *Closing the Gap in a Generation: Health Equity through Action on the Social Determinants of Health* (WHO, 2008b). The key issues, or 'principles', are as follows:

1. *Improve the conditions of daily life – the circumstances in which people are born, grow, live, work, and age.*

2. *Tackle the inequitable distribution of power, money, and resources – the structural drivers of those conditions of daily life – globally, nationally, and locally.*

3. *Measure the problem, evaluate action, expand the knowledge base, develop a workforce that is trained in the social determinants of health, and raise public awareness about the social determinants of health.*

(WHO, 2008b, p2)

In Activity 2.4, we will look at what the WHO has to say about the determinants of health in more detail.

Activity 2.4   Evidence-based practice and research

Using the link below, find the three determinants of health that the WHO identify as important.

www.who.int/hia/evidence/doh/en/

These three determinants of health are areas that we already are and will be considering in this chapter and throughout the book. Using the above link, visit the WHO website again and find the other seven factors that they consider make people healthy or not.

An outline of what you might find is given at the end of the chapter.

Following on from Activity 2.4, social and health determinants are external societal forces that have a huge influence on how well a person succeeds throughout their life course, including ill health. There is only so much the NHS (which is free healthcare at the point of access) can do if inequality in society continues. This does not mean that we, as nurses, should not do our utmost to ensure that care is delivered to a high and equitable standard. We also need to understand how social determinants affect health and that we can signpost patients for support in social care and from the multidisciplinary team.

As we have looked at these determinants from an international perspective, it is worth looking at this from a UK perspective.

Social determinants of health in the UK

The Marmot Review (Marmot et al., 2010) is a seminal report chaired by Sir Michael Marmot, moving on from chairing the WHO social determinants of health (WHO, 2008b) to focusing on the UK, taking a detailed look at social determinants of health and health inequality. The most effective way to reduce health inequalities is to make changes to the background causes of ill health, which Bell (2017) identifies as 'the accumulation of positive and negative effects of social, economic and environmental conditions on health and wellbeing throughout life' (p6). Marmot constantly identifies that improving these societal factors is the most effective way of addressing health inequality. The Marmot Review clearly acknowledges the complexities of addressing social inequalities, and so far we have highlighted that members of society from diverse and marginalised groups add an additional layer to these complexities. Government, and to a certain extent healthcare, focuses on lifestyle interventions, what the review calls 'lifestyle drift' (Marmot et al., 2010, p86). Diverse groups, such as people with learning disabilities, GTRs, migrants, asylum seekers and certain BAME populations, can belong to lower socio-economic groups that perpetuate the inequalities they face. This focus on lifestyle choices without understanding the social determinants on health makes some of these choices inevitable, such as income, housing and education. How much you earn determines where you live, and the education you attain will improve your earnings and your ability to navigate the health and social care systems to benefit your health. There is also evidence that racism is central to how the social determinants of health intersect with ethnicity, gender and mental health to reproduce social and economic inequalities within healthcare (Viruell-Fuentes et al., 2012).

As a healthcare professional, it can appear that our role will have insufficient impact on the health outcomes for diverse groups, but this is not the case. A large, knowledgeable, multidisciplinary workforce is paramount in acting on the social determinants of health. The Marmot Review clearly understands that a shortage of trained healthcare staff to deliver basic functions of service delivery, and to deliver interventions to reduce inequality and improve health outcomes, will cause a 'major impediment to success' (Marmot et al., 2010, p88). Therefore, your role is important, and it is important, as a student nurse, that you never forget this.

The life expectancy (LE) of a population gives an idea of how well it is doing regarding health. The LE of the population has increased over the past 20 years, although over recent years it has stagnated (ONS, 2019a). There also continues to be gender difference and women continue to live longer than men (ONS, 2019a). Almost all BAME groups trail the national average for life expectancy, apart from black Africans, who have the highest life expectancy for both men and women (Sunak and Rajeswaran, 2014). However, from Tables 2.4 and 2.5, you can see that for females with learning disabilities, this is not the case, and only men with mental health problems have a lower life expectancy. More comprehensive data are hard to collate as the life expectancy of different ethnic groups in a defined population has rarely been calculated due to a lack of suitable data. Where it has, substantial differences between groups have often been found, typically in favour of the ethnic majority (Gruer et al., 2016, p1253). Things are no better for the immigrant population not only with LE, but older immigrants have higher rates of chronic conditions, limitations and depression compared to their non-migrant counterparts (Reus-Pons et al., 2017). If you consider additional factors such as deprived areas, there is a life expectancy inequality gap of 6.8 years for females and 9.2 years for males, a figure that has reduced marginally from 2008 to 2012 (PHE, 2017e). These figures starkly demonstrate the continual societal forces on indicators of health.

Black African		Black Caribbean		Indian		Pakistani		Bangladeshi		Roma/gypsy	
M	F	M	F	M	F	M	F	M	F	M	F
79.83	83.17	77.1	81.8	79	82.1	77.25	80.77	77.1	81	69.2	72.9

Table 2.4 Life expectancy by ethnicity

Source: Sunak and Rajeswaran (2014, p59)

Population UK[1]		Learning disability[2]		Mental health[3]	
M	F	M	F	M	F
79.2	82.9	65.2	64.9	64.2	67.9

Table 2.5   Life expectancy of people with learning disabilities and mental health issues

Sources: (1) ONS (2017); (2) Chesney et al. (2014); (3) NHS Digital (2018)

The social influences on healthcare, as you can see, are significant, but how the government has tried to legislate against these influences that cause inequality will now be addressed.

Equality legislation

The Equality Act 2010 collated legislation that already existed covering a variety of areas and older legislation focusing on anti-discriminatory practices in work and society. Ultimately, it identified nine protected characteristics against which people cannot be discriminated. They are age, disability, gender reassignment, race, religion or belief, sex, sexual orientation, marriage and civil partnership, and pregnancy and maternity. There is a legal framework that acknowledges that discrimination exists even within a country that is so diverse.

It is important that, as healthcare professionals, we are aware that there can be legal consequences for organisations, as well as poor health outcomes for patients, if discrimination exists. The Equality Act 2010 is a good place to start looking at the different types of discrimination:

- *Direct discrimination*: This occurs when a person treats another less favourably than they treat, or would treat, others because of a protected characteristic.
- *Indirect discrimination*: This occurs when an apparently neutral policy (provision, criterion or practice) is applied 'that puts, or would put, people sharing a protected characteristic at a particular disadvantage, and puts the individual at that disadvantage' (HM Government, 2013).

Reasonable adjustment is part of the Equality Act 2010, and it is Platform 7.9 (NMC, 2018) which identifies that, as nurses, we must consider what is important and can be changed in order to ensure that when dealing with vulnerable and disabled patients, an appropriate level of care is given. An example of this in practice is that some patients require a nurse to deliver care on a one-to-one basis for the duration of their stay in hospital, or a relative can stay for long periods to be with their family member and provide essential aspects of care independently or with the assistance of a healthcare professional.

What is due regard?

Public authorities are required to have due regard of the need to eliminate unlawful discrimination, harassment and victimisation, as well as advance equality of opportunity and foster good relationships between people who share a protected characteristic and those who do not (Home Office, 2013, p7). This is further legislative indication of the importance of equality. Note that equity is not used here but as a student you are starting to interpret information in a way that benefits your patients and the care that you give.

Research summary: sex, gender and diversity

It is necessary to take a moment to think about issues of sex, gender and diversity. When looking at transgenderism and the fluidity of gender as opposed to sex, being male and female is an area that is developing and changing, and will continue to do so. In health, the biological difference of sex means that women are more likely to have breast cancer than men, but men also get breast cancer (Cancer Research UK, 2018). The Equality Act 2010 considers gender as a protected characteristic, a clear legislative acknowledgement of gender inequality. Gender is socially constructed, and the roles that men and women have in society expose them to gendered inequality; for women, this includes greater exposure to indoor air pollutants and domestic violence (O'Neill et al., 2014). Evidence repeatedly shows that BAME women report more negative experiences of maternity care, such as poor communication and a lack of empathy from healthcare professionals (Aquino et al., 2015, p374), and black women in the UK are more likely to die from complications of pregnancy and childbirth (MBRRACE-UK, 2018). Cervical cancer screening is on the decline across all women in Britain, but BAME women are more likely to be unaware of screening availability (Marlow et al., 2017). When considering intersectionality, gender is a major component that exacerbates inequality across diversity, particularly for black women (Bhopal, 2018). This does not mean that men do not have their own particular issues with healthcare. For example, men are less likely than women to seek medical help for depression, and one theory for this is their commitment to traditional masculinity – not wanting to seek help, but to carry on being 'strong' (Seidler et al., 2016).

Chapter summary

This chapter started by discussing the changing emphasis on what is considered health. It then explored crucial healthcare issues related to LD, GRT and LGBTQ communities, as well as life expectancy differences between diverse communities. The chapter introduced the term stigma and how this interacts with racism, prejudice, stereotyping and discrimination, showing how it impacts patients' experiences of healthcare, and can mean needs are not met. The importance of epidemiology and demographic genomics, as well as their effect on diverse groups, was discussed, and we built on Chapter 1's discussion on the relationship between social and health determinants and poor health outcomes for patients from diverse backgrounds. Finally, the legal framework against discrimination that exists in society and health-care was addressed by looking at the Equality Act 2010.

Activities: brief outline answers

Activity 2.1   Team-working (p26)

It is important to acknowledge the value of a positive and constructive relationship between patients, families, carers and healthcare professionals. Below is not a complete list of the MDT members that could be involved.

- *Consultant (doctor)*: LDs cover a broad spectrum of conditions; therefore, the right senior doctor is very important. Specialist knowledge, correct diagnosis and ongoing care is their role.
- *General practitioner*: Also important to the ongoing care of the patient with an LD in the community.
- *Teacher*: Education and assuring the right type of educational support for a person with an LD needs to be carefully considered due to the varied abilities that a person with an LD may have.
- *Learning disability liaison nurse*, who can help with facilitating admissions to hospital for a person with an LD, especially when it is a planned admission (RCN, 2017b, p10).
- *Community learning disability teams (CLDTs)*, who are an invaluable resource. They typically comprise of learning disability nurses, psychologists, psychiatrists, speech and language therapists, physiotherapists, occupational therapists, and arts therapists. They normally have an open referral system and are experts in helping people with learning disabilities access various community facilities, especially healthcare (RCN, 2017b).

Activity 2.2   Evidence-based practice and research (p28)

Sickle-cell anaemia

- *What ethnic groups are more likely to have the condition?* Sickle-cell disease is common in people of African, Mediterranean, Middle Eastern and Indian ancestry, and in people from the Caribbean and parts of Central and South America.
- *What is given as the reason for the genetic condition?* Being a carrier for sickle-cell disease is thought to convey some protection against malaria, and as such there is an increased prevalence of people with sickle-cell trait where malaria is common.
- *What is the clinical management of the condition?* Management guidelines recommend that all patients should receive an optimal level of care delivered close to home, as well as access to clinical experts in specialist centres. In addition, services should support 'expert' patients, parents and carers to manage the condition at home when appropriate. Multidisciplinary management should aim to prevent and treat infections, pain and complications, and include social and psycho-educational support. The mainstay of primary prevention is to avoid dehydration, extremes of temperature, physical exhaustion, and extremely high altitude.

Alpha thalassemia

- *What ethnic groups are more likely to have the condition?* Alpha thalassaemia is most prevalent in sub-Saharan Africa, South and South East Asia, the Middle East, and regions of the Mediter-ranean such as Cyprus.
- *What is given as the reason for the genetic condition?* The genetic basis of alpha thalassaemia is complex, as each person inherits two alpha-globin genes from each parent. Because of the complexity, referral to specialist clinical genetics services is recommended.

- *What is the clinical management of the condition?* Most patients with HbH disease (alpha thalassaemia) are well but will have a haematological evaluation every 6 to 12 months. Occasional red blood cell transfusions may be required, particularly during febrile illnesses when haemolytic crises are more likely.

Activity 2.3 Decision-making (p32)

From what was said in handover and by your practice supervisor considering issues of gender, ethnicity and Olufemi's sickle-cell disorder, what is being stigmatised?

The stereotype of the angry violent young black man is unfortunately a strong one, and this may dominate the interaction with you and your practice supervisor. He can be stigmatised due to having sickle-cell disease, stereotyped because of his gender and ethnicity and discriminated against. There is evidence that pain management, which is an important part of his nursing care, is not managed successfully due to stigmatisation, unconscious bias and poor clinical decision-making by healthcare professionals.

Olufemi is obviously angry. Why do you think this is?

His pain is not being managed and he is not being listened to. Previous encounters with healthcare professionals may have managed his pain inadequately, with nursing staff not knowing about how to manage his condition appropriately. This could easily lead to his behaviour. Think about how you would feel if you were in severe pain and it was not being managed in a clinical environment that should be able to manage your pain effectively.

What could you and your practice supervisor do to improve this situation?

Listen to your patient, particularly when they have a long-term condition and communicate clearly. They may well know more about their condition and how to manage it better than you, so work with them. Explain what you are doing as well as why you are doing it. Manage what is obviously his main concern – pain management. Think about why he is behaving in the way he is and look beyond your unconscious bias.

Activity 2.4 Evidence-based practice and research (p35)

Find the three determinants of health that the WHO identify as important.

1. The social and economic environment.
2. The physical environment.
3. The person's individual characteristics and behaviours.

Find the other seven factors that they consider make people healthy or not.

1. *Income and social status*: Higher income and social status are linked to better health. The greater the gap between the richest and poorest people, the greater the differences in health.
2. *Education*: Low education levels are linked with poor health, more stress and lower self-confidence.
3. *Physical environment*: Safe water and clean air, healthy workplaces, and safe houses, communities and roads all contribute to good health. Employment and working conditions – people in employment are healthier, particularly those who have more control over their working conditions.
4. *Social support networks*: Greater support from families, friends and communities is linked to better health. Culture – customs and traditions and the beliefs of the family and community all affect health.
5. *Genetics*: Inheritance plays a part in determining life span, healthiness and the likelihood of developing certain illnesses. Personal behaviour and coping skills – balanced eating, keeping active, smoking, drinking, and how we deal with life's stresses and challenges all affect health.

6. *Health services*: Access and use of services that prevent and treat disease influences health.

7. *Gender*: Men and women suffer from different types of diseases at different ages.

Further reading

Ashworth, A. (n.d.) *Sexual Orientation: A Guide for the NHS*. Available at: www.stonewall.org.uk/sites/default/files/stonewall-guide-for-the-nhs-web.pdf (accessed 20 August 2019).

Stonewall is a charity that champions the LGBTQ community in the UK and abroad, working with NHS organisations across England, helping them to meet their legal obligations, and more importantly to model best practice. Stonewall research has demonstrated that the specific needs of gay people are too often overlooked in the provision of healthcare. *Sexual Orientation: A Guide for the NHS* is a document generated by Stonewall with action plans for the NHS for LGBTQ people in England. In her foreword for this valuable report, Penny Mordaunt, Minister for Women and Equalities, outlines what was done and its importance:

> *In July 2017, the government launched a nationwide LGBT survey. The survey, which ran from July to October, asked LGBT and intersex people for their views on public services and about their experiences more generally living as a LGBT person in the UK. The survey received over 108,000 valid responses, making it the largest national survey to date of LGBT people anywhere in the world. This document provides a summary of the key findings from the survey and is useful as a healthcare professional to have an idea about the current LGBT experience in the UK.*

> (pp2–3)

EHRC (2016) *England's Most Disadvantaged Groups: Gypsies, Travellers and Roma*. Available at: http://www.equalityhumanrights.com/sites/default/files/is-england-fairer-2016-most-disadvantaged-groups-gypsies-travellers-roma.pdf (accessed 29 August 2019).

The Equality and Human Rights Commission promotes and enforces the laws that protect our rights to fairness, dignity and respect. As part of its duties, the Commission provides parliament and the nation with periodic reports on equality and human rights progress in England, Scotland and Wales. This is the first ever report on equality and human rights progress for England, highlighting the difficulties of one of the UK's most disadvantaged groups, GRTs.

Emerson, E. and Baines, S. (2011) Health inequalities and people with learning disabilities in the UK. *Tizard Learning Disability Review*, 16(1): 42–8.

This article looks at health inequalities from a learning disability perspective and writes in detail about the key areas of inequality after a substantial literature review.

Government Equalities Office (2018) *National LGBT Survey Summary Report*. Available at: https://assets.publishing.service.gov.uk/government/uploads/system/uploads/attachment_data/file/722314/GEO-LGBT-Survey-Report.pdf (accessed 20 August 2019).

In July 2017, the government launched a nationwide LGBTQ survey. The survey, which ran from July to October, asked LGBTQ and intersex people for their views on public services and about their experiences more generally living as an LGBTQ person in the UK. The survey received over 108,000 valid responses, making it the largest national survey to date of LGBTQ people anywhere in the world. This document provides a summary of the key findings from the survey, and is useful as a healthcare professional to have an idea about the current LGBTQ experience in the UK.

Healthcare Quality Improvement Partnership (HQIP) (2017) *The Learning Disabilities Mortality Review Annual Report 2017*. Available at: www.hqip.org.uk/resource/the-learning-disabilities-mortality-review-annual-report-2017/ (accessed 20 August 2019).

The Healthcare Quality Improvement Partnership (HQIP) was established in April 2008 to promote quality in healthcare and to increase the impact that clinical audit has on healthcare quality improvement. It is an independent organisation led by the Academy of

Medical Royal Colleges, the Royal College of Nursing and National Voices. The Learning Disabilities Mortality Review annual report reviews the deaths of people with learning disabilities, identifies learning from those deaths, and takes the learning forward into service improvement initiatives.

Useful websites

Learning Disability

www.learningdisability.co.uk/learning-disability/

A useful website that has valuable videos from people with learning disabilities and key points of importance when working with people with learning disabilities.

The Health Foundation

www.health.org.uk

An independent charity committed to bringing about better health and healthcare for people in the UK. They believe that good health supports positive social and economic outcomes – both for the individual and society as a whole – understanding the quality of healthcare through in-depth analysis of policy and data. To maintain and improve care while demand and costs are rising, the health and social care system needs adequate funding, a skilled workforce and increases in productivity. The Health Foundation provides evidence-based, independent comment and features on topics including NHS and social care finances, UK healthcare quality, healthcare quality improvement, and population health. This is another useful place to gather current data and analysis.

Runnymede Trust

www.runnymedetrust.org

Runnymede is a charity and the UK's leading independent race equality think tank. They generate intelligence for a multi-ethnic Britain through research, network-building, leading debate, and policy engagement. Runnymede is working to build a Britain in which all citizens and communities feel valued, enjoy equal opportunities, lead fulfilling lives, and share a common sense of belonging. They state that to effectively overcome racial inequality in society, our democratic dialogue, policy and practice should all be based on reliable evidence from rigorous research and thorough analysis. Research-based interventions are a priority in social policy and practice, and our public engagement with decision-makers will assist policymakers, practitioners and citizens to reduce the risk of our society being blighted by racism and discrimination to the detriment of us all.

Chapter 3　Diversity, communication and health literacy

Marion Hinds

NMC Standards of Proficiency for Registered Nurses

This chapter will address the following platforms and proficiencies:

Platform 1: Being an accountable professional

1.9　understand the need to base all decisions regarding care and interventions on people's needs and preferences, recognising and addressing any personal and external factors that may unduly influence their decisions.

1.11　communicate effectively using a range of skills and strategies with colleagues and people at all stages of life and with a range of mental, physical, cognitive and behavioural health challenges.

1.14　provide and promote non-discriminatory, person-centred and sensitive care at all times, reflecting on people's values and beliefs, diverse backgrounds, cultural characteristics, language requirements, needs and preferences, taking account of any need for adjustments.

Platform 2: Promoting health and preventing ill health

2.7　understand and explain the contribution of social influences, health literacy, individual circumstances, behaviours and lifestyle choices to mental, physical and behavioural health outcomes.

Chapter aims

After reading this chapter, you will be able to:

- define and explain the key terms 'health literacy' and 'communication';
- understand the relevant theory supporting the concepts of diversity, health literacy and communication, and their application to healthcare practice;

(Continued)

(Continued)

- understand the need for effective communication in order to improve health literacy in diverse groups; and
- apply knowledge and understanding to a range of work-based scenarios exploring communication and health literacy in diverse groups.

Introduction

Case study: Bernard Fitzsimmons

Bernard Fitzsimmons is a 65-year-old man who lives in a hostel for the homeless. He has had a history of weight loss, tiredness and shortness of breath, and has had a persistent cough for the past three months. His symptoms were noticed by Jacob, one of the care workers, who suggested Bernard see the visiting doctor. He was prescribed two types of medication to take. However, three weeks later, his symptoms have not improved and he is feeling worse; in particular, the cough is keeping him awake at night. Codruta, a second-year student nurse on her first community placement, accompanies the outreach nurse, Mabel, to assess Bernard at the hostel. Bernard is very quiet and looks unkempt. When Mabel questions him, his responses are a simple 'yes' or 'no' without any further details given, despite her trying to coax him to respond with more information. When Mabel leaves the room to speak with Jacob, Codruta decides to move closer to Bernard and starts by introducing herself. She asks him if he minds her talking to him; he does not look at her, but replies, 'No'. Codruta starts by asking Bernard to tell her about his life. He is hesitant at first, but slowly tells her that he became homeless after losing his job at a local factory. He then developed depression and found himself isolated and alone. Bernard continues, saying that he is very worried about his cough, but when he saw the doctor he felt hurried and the appointment was very quick. He says that he was given some tablets and does not remember being given any instructions on what to do. Bernard does not like medicines, so he did not take them and felt that he would eventually get better. He also admits that he has some difficulty with reading, writing and following information given to him, and feels embarrassed about this.

As we can see from the case study above, communication with diverse groups can be very complex. We can also see that health literacy has a significant impact upon successful health outcomes and well-being.

In this chapter, you will develop an understanding of health literacy and effective communication in relation to the care of diverse groups. Throughout this chapter, there will be activities and the application of patient scenarios from all fields of nursing, and this will enable you to appreciate the requirements and subtle differences when caring for patients from these backgrounds. Variations such as language, dialect and cultural norms are central parts of how diverse groups communicate and interact with healthcare services and must be taken into consideration during all healthcare episodes.

Over the last two decades, there has been a significant change in the demographics of the United Kingdom (UK). The diversity of groups within the population is on the increase, and this trend is set to continue, due to economic, political and environmental reasons.

For diverse groups, appropriate person-centred communication in all its forms is a key foundation in providing quality care, as well as ensuring the right access to care services. For example, the inability to engage with healthcare professionals due to issues such as limited English language skills, cognitive disability or a nomadic lifestyle, such as those in the gypsy and traveller communities, will negatively impact on the maintenance of optimum health. There are many reasons why challenges arise when communicating with diverse groups, and these will be discussed in this chapter. It is important that, as a nurse, you are alert to these.

Literacy is the capability to read, write, speak, listen and understand written communication to an appropriate level that enables us to function well in society and to make sense of the world in which we live (National Literacy Trust, 2017). In England, one in seven people (i.e. 5.1 million people) are deficient in basic literacy skills (Department for Business, Innovation and Skills, 2012). In a diverse and often marginalised group, such as those belonging to the gypsy, Roma and traveller communities, low literacy levels are commonplace. In a recent report by Scadding and Sweeney (2018), it is noted that in this age of increasing digital communication, there is a significant reduction in the ability of these communities to access and use computer technology. The 2011 census has also highlighted the high number of gypsy or Irish travellers in England and Wales between the ages of 16 and 24 and over 65 who have no academic or professional qualifications, in comparison to their peers in the rest of the country.

The term 'health literacy' is defined by Public Health England as 'people having the appropriate skills, knowledge and confidence to access, understand, evaluate, use and navigate health and social care information and services' (PHE, 2015b, p5). Health literacy is the clear communication and correct understanding of health information, according to Osborne (2013). The Nursing and Midwifery Council standards (NMC, 2018) define health literacy as 'the degree to which individuals can obtain, process, and understand basic health information and services needed to make appropriate health decisions' (p35). Health literacy can be divided into three categories:

1. *Functional health literacy*: This is described as the basic level of reading, writing, numeracy and discussion skills that an individual will need to function effectively in daily life.

2. *Communicative/interactive health literacy:* It is important for individuals to have skills that equip them with the ability to distinguish what information is important and relevant. This will, in turn, help them to make good and effective health decisions.

3. *Critical health literacy:* This is about an individual having greater control over their life by using the skill of critical analysis when sourcing information. This includes areas such as the promotion of health and well-being and the self-management of their own conditions.

The Royal College of General Physicians produced a report on health literacy in recognition of the need for patients and the public to understand and act upon health information (RCGP, 2014). This means that healthcare professionals must recognise the importance of patients having adequate health literacy skills during healthcare interactions.

In order to deliver care that is inclusive and sensitive to diverse patient needs, consideration has to be given to the way in which the multidisciplinary team communicate in clinical practice. Effective communication is the cornerstone for all fields of nursing practice, and is one of the ways in which compassion, sensitivity and caring can be conveyed in order to promote collaboration and cooperation in the clinical setting (Bloomfield and Pegram, 2015; Crawford et al., 2015). Compassion in Practice (Department of Health, 2012a) highlighted the importance of the 6 Cs, which are care, compassion, competence, communication, courage and commitment. These are fundamental nursing skills that may be more challenging to achieve when working with diverse groups. The National Health Service (NHS) is the foundation of healthcare provision and reflects a system that will offer treatment to all, which implies equity and justice. You will now have knowledge of some key terms that are used when exploring the subject of health literacy. The next section will provide you with information on self-awareness and how it can negatively and positively influence your interactions with patients.

Self-awareness

As a student, you will come across patients from all walks of life and from a wide range of backgrounds. The Nursing and Midwifery Council code of conduct for nurses and midwives (NMC, 2015) makes clear that in prioritising people, the nurse or midwife will 'avoid making assumptions and recognise diversity and individual choice' (p4). This calls for tolerance and acceptance of others, even if you do not understand their particular way of life. This should not affect the care that you provide. As a student nurse, you will need to develop the skill of self-awareness to know and understand yourself in order to understand and relate to others (Jack and Smith, 2007).

As individuals, we have values and beliefs that stem from our upbringing, social class, environment, culture and experiences in life that we see as normal (Jasper, 2003). However, we must appreciate that these same values and beliefs may not be seen as normal to others.

An appreciation of self-awareness enables us to consciously recognise characteristics about ourselves, and these can be strengths or weaknesses. This recognition will enable us to be more readily available to help others (Burnard, 1992). As a registered nurse, you are required to act as a role model to others. This means that your attitude and behaviour will be observed by many people, including patients when you are in clinical practice. If you do not have an understanding of self-awareness and the way in which you portray yourself, not only can you cause offence, but your ability to develop effective interactions with patients will be limited.

As a student, you must avoid making assumptions based upon inaccurate information about cultural differences. This is known as stereotyping and can lead us to be less accommodating when dealing with patients. Stereotyping can be described as a simplistic and generalised view of a group, person or thing. The concept can be positive or negative (Stangor, 2009); unfortunately, both can be detrimental. Some examples of stereotypical views include 'elderly patients need a lot of nursing care', 'black people are good at sports', 'single mothers rely on benefits', 'women are caring', 'men are aggressive', and 'travellers are unscrupulous in business dealings', which you should appreciate are generalised descriptions of these groups. By stereotyping people, we limit our ability to form worthwhile therapeutic relationships with patients. Our behaviour may therefore be negatively influenced during our interactions with them. Unfortunately, we then neglect to take into account the uniqueness of each person with whom we come into contact. The more nurses gain exposure and interaction with others from diverse groups, the more experience and understanding will be gained. As a student nurse, you will have a range of transferable skills as well as knowledge that can be applied in your day-to-day practice.

The following scenario provides an example of how life experience and self-awareness can potentially influence a patient admission in the clinical setting.

Scenario: Hospital admission of a learning disability service user

Michael is a third-year learning disability nursing student who has just started placement on an adult surgical assessment ward. He is working with his practice assessor, Kamala, who is currently admitting 18-year-old Simon who lives in a care home. He has autism and is able to make himself understood. Simon is accompanied by a carer, Janet, who says that Simon has abdominal pain but that she does not know anything more. Simon appears quiet and withdrawn and does not make eye contact; he is also groaning intermittently. Kamala is finding the situation challenging as there is limited information available and she is becoming frustrated as Simon is reluctant to communicate. Michael is confident in his experience in situations such as this due to his training so far. He also has a younger brother with autism but has never talked to anyone at work about this. He would like to talk to Simon but feels reluctant to do so.

As you can see from this scenario, there are a number of aspects to think about in terms of using appropriate and effective communication strategies when caring for Simon.

Activity 3.1 now asks you some questions in relation to the scenario about Simon.

Activity 3.1   Reflection

After reading the above scenario, consider the following questions:

- How do you think Simon might be feeling?
- Why do you think Michael is feeling reluctant to intervene, and what should he do in this situation?

You can read underpinning information on the concept of learning disability below.

An outline answer to the scenario can be found at the end of the chapter.

The government White Paper *Valuing People* (Department of Health, 2001) identified that individuals with learning disabilities are among 'the most vulnerable and socially excluded in our society' (p2), and 'substantial health care needs are often unmet' and they are 'likely to have greater health needs' (p6). The term 'learning disability' encompasses a wide range of conditions that can be classified as mild, moderate, severe or profound, and occurs when the brain is in the developmental phase (Taylor, 2015). According to Mencap (n.d.), 'A learning disability is a reduced intellectual ability and difficulty with everyday activities – for example household tasks, socialising or managing money – which affects someone for their whole life'. When communicating with an individual who has a learning disability, healthcare professionals should first and foremost view the person rather than the impairment. Assumptions should never be made about the level of intellect the individual possesses.

The next scenario will highlight an example of an interaction with a health professional and a mother and her child from a diverse group. Communication with children and parents will require skills and knowledge of child development and learning ability, as well as any diverse group considerations. In terms of traveller identity, the umbrella definition is used for those populations originating from a nomadic cultural background, which includes Romany, Welsh, English, Roma and fairground communities (RCGP, 2013). Challenges include the regular movement of these groups, and therefore continued and regular access to healthcare services can be sporadic. Levels of literacy tend to be low and there may be widespread beliefs in self-care practices that will reduce health outcomes and limit collaboration with healthcare professionals (RCGP, 2013). Read the scenario below, which concerns a health consultation between a traveller mother, her child and the diabetes nurse specialist.

Scenario: Health consultation with a mother and child

Selina is a 9-year-old girl who was diagnosed with diabetes a year ago. Her family are travellers and they tend to move around the country quite frequently. Since this diagnosis, the family have remained in the local area. She lives with her mother, father and four brothers in a mobile home. Selina is having a consultation with Lucia, the diabetes nurse specialist, regarding the stabilisation of her condition. There have been ongoing challenges in the management of her blood glucose levels. Selina attends the local primary school, and she is very sociable and energetic. She loves to be outdoors and belongs to a number of local activity groups, such as swimming and dance. Selina has attended the appointment with her mother, who is very anxious about this meeting, and keeps stating that she 'does not know why this has happened to Selina'. Lucia is aware from previous encounters that Selina's mother has only recently come around to accepting her daughter's condition. More recently, Selina has been complaining that she is very tired.

In situations such as those described above, communication can be hindered by specific health beliefs that are held by the parties involved. This calls for sensitivity by the nurse towards both Selina and her mother in order to facilitate effective person-centred care.

Activity 3.2 asks you to think about the situation presented in the above scenario about Selina.

Activity 3.2   Communication and decision-making

What issues concerning Selina and her health need to be considered?

What can be done to help Selina's mother cope better with the current situation?

An outline answer can be found at the end of the chapter.

Continuing on with the importance of communication between healthcare professionals and patients, the following case study provides a stark illustration of the implications of poor health literacy and communication breakdown, the circumstances of which involved a young mother, a father and their newborn baby.

Case study: Significant failure of communication

In July 2009, a 21-year-old woman gave birth to a healthy baby boy at a local general hospital. The parents were Tamil refugees from Sri Lanka and the mother spoke only

(Continued)

(Continued)

a few words of English. Two days later, mother and baby were discharged from the hospital in the early afternoon but could not leave until approximately eight hours later when the father and a friend who spoke better English were coming to collect them. By this time, the baby was continuously crying; however, the mother was told by the midwives that this was normal behaviour in newborns. The father had asked if mother and baby could remain in hospital another two days, when he would be off work and more able to assist at home, but was told this was not possible. When the father and friend arrived, the friend questioned if the discharge should go ahead as the baby was crying, but was told it was normal. The friend and parents took the baby to the car and again returned to ask if a doctor could look at the baby, but were told again that crying was normal. They were advised that if anything was wrong, they could bring the baby back. The community midwife arrived at 12.40 p.m. the next day to the couple's home and found the baby 'pale, lethargic and not interested in feeding' (Dyer, 2018, p1). The baby had not been fed since more than 15 hours earlier and there was no milk formula in the house. An ambulance was called; however, the baby 'was in a hypoglycaemic state' (Dyer, 2018, p1), which caused severe, catastrophic brain injuries.

The child now has cerebral palsy and severe physical and cognitive impairment. Failings were found in terms of poor communication engagement with the mother due to language barriers. Unfortunately, this was a poor discharge as opportunities for a safe discharge outcome, such as the use of an interpreter to facilitate better communication with the mother, were missed. The judge ruled that if the baby had been checked before the family left the hospital, the outcome would have been avoided. It was acknowledged that the mother had attempted to voice her concerns, but due to the language barrier she could not make herself understood. As such, no information had been provided to the parents in relation to the necessity of feeding their newborn baby. Additionally, the provision of information from staff that could be easily understood by the parents was not demonstrated in this tragic case.

As the above case study clearly demonstrates, skilled engagement with individuals from diverse backgrounds requires the consideration of certain nuances, terminology and norms of which the healthcare professional may not know about. It is therefore necessary that, as a student nurse, you develop effective, purposeful, person-centred communication skills to successfully perform in your current and future role as a registered nurse. Another key component of this process is the ability to facilitate an appropriate level of engagement with the patient in order to enable a responsive and meaningful therapeutic relationship. Diverse groups with linguistic needs must be recognised and appropriate care delivered; nurses 'must learn how to interact with and care for patients' (Coulter, 2011, p143). According to McDonald (2016), the estimated cost of poor communication to the NHS is more than £1 billion per year. Patients need to feel that they are able to trust the healthcare professional caring for them to be mindful and anticipatory of their needs. Effective communication is clearly linked to patient safety.

From reading this chapter so far, you will have an idea of the necessity for good communication skills and what can happen if this does not occur. The next section will discuss in more detail communication and health literacy as applied to diverse groups.

Communication and health literacy in diverse groups

Communication is central to successful caring relationships and effective team working. Listening is as important as what we say and do. It is essential for 'no decision about me, without me'. Communication is the key to a good workplace with benefits for those in our care and staff alike.

(NHS England, 2012, p13)

Before continuing to read the rest of the chapter, take some time to complete Activity 3.3.

Activity 3.3 Research and reflection

Write down your own definition of the word 'communication' and the different types you can find.

Look up two definitions of the word 'communication'. What are the similarities and in what ways do they differ?

Make a list of the different ways in which individuals may communicate.

What strategies would you use in order to communicate with someone who did not share the same language as you?

There is no model answer at the end of the chapter as this is based on your own reflections; however, the next section provides some outline answers to the questions.

Having thought about the issues raised in Activity 3.3, it is apparent that, as a nurse, communication is possibly the most important skill that is required when dealing with patients. The process involves the whole being and is at the heart of the delivery of quality nursing care. It is the foundation upon which we develop and maintain relationships, and there are certain ethical, legal and professional implications for nurses. However, communication is of no use if the recipient is unable to understand and act upon the information being given. As human beings, we each communicate in a number of ways and by various methods. Good communication will depend upon the skill of the health professional to deliver a clear message to the patient (Kourkouta and Papathanasiou, 2014).

Communication may be simply defined as the interactive passage or passing of information between parties – sender and receiver – using means such as writing, speaking or the use of a common sign system of behaviour (Ali, 2017; Bach and Grant, 2015). More recently, the use of email and social media is becoming increasingly popular, which adds to both the ease and complexity of communicating. According to the Department of Health (2010a), communication is 'a process that involves a meaningful exchange between at least two people to convey facts, needs, opinions, thoughts, feelings or other information through verbal and non-verbal means, including face-to-face exchanges and the written word' (p95).

However, if you think about the process of communication, you will appreciate that it can be fraught with difficulty, as once something is said it cannot be taken back; in other words, it is irreversible. Another definition is that communication is the 'imparting or exchanging of information by speaking, writing, or using some other medium' (Lexico, 2019a). You may find that when exploring the definition of the word 'communication', there are more similarities than differences. Examples of similarities may include:

- The process involves more than one person, and those involved will take on the role of sender or receiver, and these roles can interchange during the communication interaction.
- Communication is also dependent upon the context or circumstances in which the process takes place.
- An integral part of the process is that those involved will understand the messages being passed between each other.
- There are numerous influences that can enhance and disrupt the communication process.
- The purpose of communication models is to explain the complexity of communication theory.

A key difference in communication definitions may be found in the wording used to describe the term. There are also subtle differences in the components that make up theoretical models such as the transactional model of communication, which is described on pages 55–7.

Groups tend to share common verbal and non-verbal ways in which initial greetings are made when meeting with others (e.g. the spoken word or the use of body language, such as a handshake, nod or smile). Each individual will attach specific meaning to these responses.

Two key characteristics of the communication process are the message being sent and the relationship between those involved. The quality and value of the communication process is strongly linked to patient satisfaction and positive patient experiences. As a student, you need to be mindful of individual patient behaviour during the health and illness continuum. The presentation and experience of signs and symptoms in areas such as pain and anxiety can alter the communication process (Bloomfield and Pegram, 2015; Peacock and Patel, 2008). The NMC (2018) makes clear that, as a nurse, you are to 'provide and promote non-discriminatory, person-centred and sensitive care at all times, reflecting on people's values and beliefs, diverse backgrounds, cultural characteristics, language requirements, needs and preferences, taking account of any need for adjustments' (p9).

Communication with patients can be problematic for a number of reasons, the most important being an assumption that the information delivered is understood and will be appropriately acted upon. For diverse and often vulnerable groups, there will be additional unique differences, such as culture, linguistic needs, income, socio-economic position and cognitive ability, and these can adversely impact upon their access and engagement with healthcare services. The global emergence of health literacy as a concept is borne out of this and the recognition that health literacy is a significant determinant of health status (RCGP, 2014; WHO, 2013).

Health literacy is relevant during all stages of the life continuum, and a lack of key literate skills will negatively impact an individual's life from childhood to adulthood. Many people function adequately with low literacy skills and illiteracy and never disclose their limitation. There is no way to distinguish if a person has a low level of literacy, and educational achievement is not a reliable indicator. The link between shame and health literacy has been explored by Parikh et al. (1996). This study found that nearly 40 per cent of patients who acknowledged trouble reading admitted they felt shame. A significant number of respondents had not told their spouses or their children. In terms of screening for literacy ability, this also accompanies negative feelings of shame (Wolf et al., 2007). This topic was identified at the beginning of this chapter in the case study about Bernard Fitzsimmons.

As a nurse, you need to ensure that you deal sensitively with issues of literacy. Signs of low literacy include the patient asking very few or no questions, non-compliance with medications, and the inability to provide a coherent history of complaints and complete forms. In addition to regular missed appointments, the identification of medications by sight (rather than reading labels), and being unable to explain their prescribed medications.

A report published by the National Literacy Trust confirmed that 'people with low levels of literacy are more likely to live in deprived communities, be financially worse off, and have poorer health' (Gilbert et al., 2018, p3). In addition, the same study found significant differences in life expectancy between geographical areas and within communities with the poorest literacy by as much as 26 years (male) and 20 years (female). Those with weak health literacy are at more risk of hospital admission and less likely to use preventative services or manage their health conditions well (PHE, 2015b). Literacy has an impact upon people's ability to access and use information. This further confirms the need to address the health literacy needs of diverse populations.

Another key terminology when considering health literacy is mental health literacy (MHL), which is defined as the 'knowledge and beliefs about mental disorders which aid their recognition, management or prevention' (Jorm et al., 1997). It is possible to conclude that if an individual experiences life-affecting psychological symptoms, they will attempt to manage the symptoms. Therefore, symptom management strategies, such as seeking support from family and friends, will be influenced by their own level of mental health literacy (Jorm, 2000).

Public Health England identify that policymakers at the local and government level must collaborate with the health and social care sectors, including schools, employers and adult education services, to address the health literacy agenda (PHE, 2015b).

In the next scenario about Lazarus, you will be able to explore the concept of mental health literacy further.

Scenario: Mental health literacy

Lazarus is a 24-year-old African Caribbean man who was diagnosed with schizophrenia three years previously. Initially, he was not accepting of his condition, and this led to his non-compliance with medication therapy. He was admitted to an acute mental health ward for assessment and further management. He is now stabilised and lives in social housing accommodation, and Imran is his assigned key worker. Lazarus has close ties with his mother and father and visits them daily, often staying over if he does not feel like going home. His mother is very involved with his condition and ongoing care. One evening while he is watching television, his mother notices a plaster on his arm and asks him what has happened. Lazarus tells her that he received a call earlier in the day to attend an appointment with Basil, the mental health nurse, and a blood test was taken. Lazarus has no idea why. His mother is very upset that he is unable to give her any further information and plans to call Basil the next day to find out what is going on.

Take time to reflect on what you have read so far on health and mental health literacy before continuing with Activity 3.4.

Activity 3.4   Reflection and critical thinking

What do you consider are the issues with Lazarus?

What do you think could be done to help Lazarus?

What information would you give to Lazarus's mother?

An outline answer can be found at the end of the chapter.

The issue of mental health literacy is one of growing importance given the increase of individuals experiencing mental health problems in society. The key aim of the

National Service Framework for Mental Health (1999) is to achieve equality and combat discrimination for individuals and groups experiencing mental health difficulties. Disparities have been identified in the ability to access services among black, Asian and minority ethnic (BAME) groups, which will have a negative outcome on overall well-being. A study carried out by Memon et al. (2016) on perceived barriers to accessing mental health services by BAME communities in the south of England concluded a number of key areas that required attention. The 'inability to recognise and accept mental health problems' was cited as a key issue (p1). Language barriers and poor communication were factors that affected relationships between the parties involved. Additionally, men were found to be a 'hard-to-reach group' and 'were more reluctant to seek help and felt excluded' from services (p7). The study also identified that the responsiveness of services to the diverse needs of BAME service users was limited.

In the next section, we will look at the theoretical basis of a specific communication model and types of communication, such as non-verbal and interpersonal, as well as the use of interpreter services.

The transactional model of communication

A knowledge-based foundation of communication theory is important for effective nursing practice. The use of a communication model will provide information on the stages of the process and is often graphically represented. However, while this will detail the different aspects, it may not provide the reader with a conscious idea of the multiple complexities involved during the process.

The transactional model of communication developed by Wood in 2004 considers the fact that numerous channels of communication exist during face-to-face interactions. The model also proposes that those involved both send and receive messages simultaneously and are identified as 'communicators'. Wood (2006) defines communication as a 'systemic process in which people interact with and through symbols to create and interpret meanings' (p503). The term 'symbol' in this context is pertinent as it denotes a meaning that will vary between people. The model is one that is easily applied to communication with diverse groups as it incorporates how the areas of social, relational and cultural context make up and influence our communication interactions (Anonymous, 2016). Simply put, the model takes note of the interpersonal aspects of communication as well as the spoken word. It is recognised that outside or external interference, known as noise, as well as internal dialogue, will have an effect on the interaction. External noise, for example, may include a patient pressing a call bell in another area of the ward or a telephone ringing. Internal noise might involve the subjective feeling of anger or tiredness in either participant during the communication process.

The model theorises that during this constant flow of verbal and non-verbal messages that pass back and forth between those involved, we are able to construct and revise our communication during the encounter based upon the messages received.

The channels of communication will include nuances such as body angle, presentation, tone of voice and role portrayal (Pavord and Donnelly, 2015). The reaction of each participant during the communication episode will depend upon factors such as cultural beliefs, previous experience, attitude and background.

As identified, a lack of patient engagement with healthcare systems and processes will inevitably lead to inadequacies and reduced patient satisfaction. Communication cannot be escaped from, and, as a student nurse, you must develop the skills to take note, interpret and understand the information provided by the patient. This can be clearly demonstrated in the nursing process. The collection of accurate information through meaningful dialogue with the patient by the use of verbal and non-verbal means will allow for the development of an effective care plan.

A holistic assessment will provide a robust foundation upon which to identify and prioritise relevant nursing problems, goals and appropriate interventions to address health needs (Ballantyne, 2016). McCarthy et al. (2013) conducted a study among undergraduate student nurses that explored the issues faced when communicating with patients who did not share the same first language. A number of concerns were raised about the students' ability to perform an accurate and comprehensive patient assessment, the effective use of translator services, and the interpretation of non-verbal cues. If you consider the assessment process, for example, it is important to develop a rapport with the patient; if not, this can result in a lack of information that can have a detrimental effect on health outcomes. This further reinforces the complexity and challenge of developing sound communication strategies with others in our care.

The Essence of Care benchmarks for communication place emphasis upon 'the specific needs, wants and preferences of people and carers' (Department of Health, 2010a, p90). The document makes clear that patients and service users must be given ample opportunity to communicate with healthcare providers, and aids, such as books, toys, large print, braille and the use of an interpreter, should be employed where necessary. An initial and ongoing assessment of communication needs will be carried out for the duration of the patient or service user contact. There is a requirement for healthcare professionals to demonstrate effective interpersonal skills and communicate with each other to formulate a collaborative plan of patient care.

Activity 3.5 asks you to access the communication benchmark and examine your own practice in conjunction with the agreed outcomes.

Activity 3.5   Communication and reflection

Read the Essence of Care benchmarks for communication, which can be downloaded from the link below.

https://assets.publishing.service.gov.uk/government/uploads/system/ uploads/attachment_data/file/216695/dh_119973.pdf

Consider your own nursing practice. In what ways are you able to demonstrate achievement of the agreed patient-focused outcomes on pages 8 and 9 of the document?

If you are unable to show that you can achieve the outcomes, what action will you take in order to do so?

As these answers are based on your own thoughts and experiences, there is no outline answer at the end of the chapter. Strategies to achieve successful outcomes can be found in the relevant Essence of Care document.

The Compassion in Practice strategy (Department of Health, 2012a) includes communication as a key area for action. A study conducted by Norouzinia et al. (2016) on communication barriers identified that reluctance by nurses to communicate was highlighted by patients as one of the most frequent complaints. The study concluded that the best way to achieve patient satisfaction was through effective and appropriate communication. A study conducted by Taylor et al. (2013) investigated inter-professional views of caring for ethnic minorities with limited or no English speaking skills. Their findings, under the theme 'barriers of cross-cultural communication', concluded that aspects such as language barriers, low literacy, health beliefs and lack of understanding negatively influenced the hospital experience.

Verbal communication

The NMC (2018) makes clear the requirement of a nurse or midwife to:

communicate effectively using a range of skills and strategies with colleagues and people at all stages of life and with a range of mental, physical, cognitive and behavioural health challenges.

(p1)

provide and promote non-discriminatory, person-centred and sensitive care at all times, reflecting on people's values and beliefs, diverse backgrounds, cultural characteristics, language requirements, needs and preferences, taking account of any need for adjustments.

(p1)

Verbal communication, simply put, is the use of the spoken word to participate in a mutual exchange with another. The purpose of this process is to convey and impart information, and will involve attention to the native language, dialect and local variations in use by the patient. It would be unreasonable to expect you, as a student, to be familiar with every aspect of verbal communication style in respect of the individuals you come into contact with. However, to purposefully engage with patients, there must be some development of meaningful exchange in order to encourage open dialogue and trust. Argyle et al. (1970) deduced that during a face-to-face interaction, only 7 per cent of a message is made up of words; 55 per cent is body language, with tone, syntax and tempo making up the remaining 38 per cent. Given that such a small percentage is focused upon the verbal transmission of information, this demonstrates the significant relevance of non-verbal communication. As good practice, try to remember this fact when you next interact with someone whose first language is not English.

The use of interpreter services

When communicating with individuals who have limited or no understanding of the English language, every effort must be made to secure the services of an interpreter. LanguageLine is a telephone interpretation service that is most frequently used in the UK. If this is not available, then the physical presence of an interpreter has to be employed in order to facilitate an appropriate level of dialogue (Bloomfield and Pegram, 2015). Assistance from a family member or friend should not be considered unless there is no alternative option, it is an emergency situation, or at the patient's request. This must not be normal practice as there is the possibility of passing inaccurate or false information to or on behalf of the patient; in addition, there may be safeguarding implications (Pavord and Donnelly, 2015). The potential to cause harm and compromise safety is increased if there is mistranslation, a breakdown in communication, or no communication at all (McClimens et al., 2014). This is clearly demonstrated in the scenario on Lazarus on page 54.

The environment where the communication is to take place should be quiet, away from any disturbances, and the process should not be rushed. The participants should consist only of those who are directly involved, and seating should be arranged in a way that is inclusive and allows for direct communication with the patient, interpreter and health professional. The health professional must check with the patient as to how they would like to be addressed and introductions made so that the patient is aware of the roles of those present, as well as the purpose of the communication. Speech should be appropriately pitched and paced when speaking to the patient, without the use of complex terminology or jargon, to allow for easy interpretation. If possible, written information should be provided in the native-language format, and the use of pictures, signs and symbols can be used to further enhance the patient's understanding. Information provided to the patient should be repeated as often as necessary during the communication process.

Burnham et al. (2008) developed the acronym 'social grraacceess' to assist professionals in the development of their self-awareness skills when working with a range of differences in individuals. As a student, it is recommended that as good practice, you use reflection to develop your knowledge and understanding. Try to think about each of the concepts listed below when you come into contact with patients:

- **G**ender
- **R**ace
- **R**eligion
- **A**ge
- **A**bility
- **C**lass
- **C**ulture
- **E**thnicity
- **E**ducation
- **S**exuality
- **S**pirituality

Before reading further, complete Activity 3.6, which asks you to consider these terms in more detail.

Activity 3.6 Research and critical thinking

Access relevant resources to find a definition and make your own notes on each of the terms in the above acronym, 'social grraacceess'.

Definitions for each can be found in the content of this book so will not be provided as an answer at the end of the chapter.

The previous section explored a communication model, verbal communication and the use of interpreter services. You should now have a better understanding of the relevance of these components in promoting positive patient–nurse interactions.

The next part of this chapter will examine the components of non-verbal communication, which is necessary given that the majority of our communication is conducted through non-verbal means.

Interpersonal communication

The 'interpersonal nature of communication' gives specific focus to the way in which two or more individuals or groups are involved and 'behave towards and feel about one another' (Bach and Grant, 2015, p14). As a student, you will be involved with patients in varied settings, such as the patient's home, clinics and the ward, and many issues will require consideration during these interactions. Interpersonal skills are considered a sound basis for professional practice and the development of a patient-centred relationship based upon trust, respect, and compassion and understanding (Bloomfield and Pegram, 2015). There are many facets to interpersonal communication, and, as a nurse, you must develop the ability to set aside prejudice, bias and stereotyping (Bach and Grant, 2015) and place focus upon the individual.

Non-verbal communication

Non-verbal communication is that which is without words, or the use of wordless cues and features such as touch, eye contact, proximity and head movement. Use of body language, posture, odour and facial expressions are considered non-verbal expressions of communication (Pavord and Donnelly, 2015). It is important to bear in mind that non-verbal communication is just as powerful as other forms, if not more so, as profound meaning can be transmitted by gestures and even silence (Ali, 2018). In terms of diverse groups, this form of communication can prove challenging, and this is because, as nurses, we may not be conversant with certain cultural expressions, which can lead to misunderstandings in our dealings with patients from diverse groups in our care. Nurses must also be aware of their body language (e.g. a nurse who appears to be very busy may be perceived by the patient as unapproachable, so care may be delayed, which may result in negative consequences). Judgements are made about a person's appearance, and it is important that, as a student, you do not make unsound speculation about others in your care.

Good listening skills demonstrate that you are interested in those who you are relating to, and at times can be hard to achieve. When listening, you should give the speaker your undivided attention, focus on the words being spoken, and try not to interrupt. In the delivery of nursing care, it is important that you ask for clarification if there is something said that you do not understand – ask the patient or service user for clarification. It is necessary that you maintain an open mind so that you can be receptive to patients and service users. With practice, listening skills can be developed, and, as a student, during your work on the ward, try to find ways in which to improve this skill. Listening is not just about silence, but involves verbal and non-verbal responses (Benbow and Jordan, 2016).

Eye contact or gaze can be an indication of the level of attention being paid to the speaker, and vice versa, and plays a vital role in social interactions (McCarthy et al., 2006). Imagine if you were speaking with someone and their gaze was elsewhere – your cultural background would play a key part in your interpretation of the situation. In Western society, it is polite to give eye contact and a sign that you may have something to hide if you do not. In West African culture, it is considered a sign of disrespect for young people to directly gaze into the eyes of an older person (elder). Knowledge or discussion with the patient or service user will be necessary so as not to mistakenly cause any offence.

The use of touch during communication enhances the encounter, but only when appropriate (e.g. in the delivery of physical care). In some circumstances, such as communicating bad news, while touch might seem appropriate, it might not be to the recipient (Pavord and Donnelly, 2015). Touch is linked to the demonstration of empathy, and offers a physical connection to another, but must be used with caution. Each communication encounter with individuals from diverse groups is unique. If the nurse has any doubts about the appropriateness of touch, it is better to withhold this gesture until certain, so as not to cause any offence. In line with touch is the proximity of one individual to another, also known as personal space. There are differences in terms of our distance between others (e.g. travelling on public transportation in rush hour, you will more than likely be in very close proximity to – or even touching – another person). Nurses must ensure that they are mindful that some patients and service users from diverse groups may not appreciate close proximity. Situations will differ, and if we are engaged with personal care activities or supporting a patient where close distance is necessary, understanding that this might not be comfortable or agreeable to some individuals is necessary. In situations such as these, attention must be paid to the non-verbal responses a patient or service user may convey.

Body language is a powerful tool and aids the communication process. People communicate continuously; even our type of dress or the way we sit or position ourselves will send a message to others. Aspects such as age, gender and social position can influence the communication process in a positive or negative manner.

Consider the scenario in Activity 3.7, which you may well encounter at some stage in your practice. This provides a typical example of the need to recognise and, insofar as possible, accurately interpret a patient's body language during interactions.

Activity 3.7   Communication and reflection

Imagine that yourself and another nurse are in the process of turning a patient who is bed-bound and speaks limited English. You notice that the patient has her eyes closed; she is grimacing and squeezing your hand.

What are your thoughts about how the patient might be feeling?

Imagine the same scenario, but this time the patient has her eyes open and is smiling at you.

What are your thoughts now about how the patient might be feeling?

An outline answer is provided at the end of the chapter.

The chapter will continue by discussing two further areas of the communication process, namely intrapersonal communication and paralanguage.

Intrapersonal communication

Intrapersonal communication requires us to know ourselves and is the form of communication that takes place within us on a constant basis (Pavord and Donnelly, 2015). This form of internal dialogue enables us to think, feel and recollect on certain narratives and enables learning to take place. Reflection is a tool that enables us to break down and examine situations and experiences that are encountered within and outside of practice. As nurses, reflection is a key component of the learning process, and according to Price (2017), 'reflective practice is at the centre of nursing' (p53). To engage in a process of self-reflection allows for professional growth and development in terms of understanding who we are (Jack and Smith, 2007), as well as those around us.

Paralanguage

Paralanguage is that which refers to accent, speed of the spoken word, tone and pitch, which have considerable negative and positive implications when communicating with diverse groups. Put simply, it is the way in which we pitch our tone and speak with particular emphasis upon certain words, which will change the meaning of the sentence. The delivery of a simple sentence can cause a breakdown in the nurse–patient relationship, as well as causing distress and anxiety to the patient. As explained by Richardson (2017), 'paralanguage makes clear what the meaning is' (p30). It is an attempt to 'understand the mood or emotional state of the person' (p30). However, paralanguage in certain groups may be misunderstood and lead to stereotyping and bias. An example of this is the 'angry black woman', as discussed by Ashley (2014) against the backdrop of mental health issues. In this paper, she identifies and explores the negativity surrounding personal descriptors used to explain behaviour apparently exhibited by black women. Terms such as 'aggressive', 'ignorant', 'hostile' and 'ill-tempered' do nothing to dispel the myths that further compound the negative stereotyping towards a specific group of people. In order to deliver care to diverse groups, account must be taken of individual differences so that patients are not subjected to negative interactions, and therefore poorer health outcomes.

Many barriers exist that can hinder the development of effective communication during the nurse–patient relationship. The next section will provide a summary of those barriers associated with communication among diverse groups, some of which have been highlighted throughout this chapter.

Communication barriers and diverse groups

Activity 3.8 asks you to think about possible barriers to the communication process.

Activity 3.8   Reflection

Make a list of as many communication barriers that you can think of and/or those you may have observed in clinical practice.

You may find that the barriers can be separated into categories such as nurse, patient or environmental-related factors.

Suggest one solution for each barrier example you have listed.

There is no outline answer at the end of the chapter, but some possible answers to the questions above are provided in the next section.

As identified in your reading so far, communication with diverse groups within the UK population is worthy of in-depth consideration given the complexities that may arise. Coupled with this are the potential barriers that may be encountered during the communication process, some of which are listed below.

Environment

As a nurse, you must be mindful of the type and purpose of the discussion when considering where meetings should take place. Any discussion involving sensitive information should preferably take place in a quiet room with minimal disruptions. If not, then a quiet area must be found; failure to do so might negatively impact the quality of the communication process. Prior to the meeting, the nurse should be aware of who will be present and that the patient concerned is in agreement to the presence of others.

Emotional

Patients will experience a range of emotions during the communication process, and these can include anger, fear, sadness, anxiety, grief and shame, dependent upon the specific circumstances. Allow sufficient time for the patient to convey their feelings. The use of silence and pauses during the discussion may help to alleviate the level of emotion experienced by the patient. The experience of the nurse involved is also relevant, as highlighted later in this section.

Professional barriers

These include aspects such as limited resources, lack of time, increased workload capacity, staff conflict and fatigue, all of which can affect the communication process. While some of these may not easily be within your control, as a nurse, you must develop an awareness of any adverse effects that may hinder the quality of your interaction with patients.

Language barriers

As identified earlier in the chapter, the use of interpreter services is strongly advised to prevent any communication breakdown or miscommunication. For example, in some diverse groups, there may be no specific word in their language to clarify certain feelings. Therefore, patience and encouragement are required to obtain accurate information, particularly if there is an issue with the level of patient literacy. If appropriate, the use of pictures or symbols may help to increase the level of understanding.

Relationship dynamics

The importance of the dynamics of the people involved in the communication process must not be underestimated, and will include the patient, nurse and any other member of the multidisciplinary team. A lack of understanding will lead to poor patient engagement and comprehension. Previous poor experience with healthcare professionals will impact on subsequent interactions, which can negatively influence patient understanding, compliance and adherence to the information provided. In some diverse groups, individuals may not see themselves as equal partners in relation to their healthcare needs. As a nurse, you must recognise the relevance of equality and collaborate with the patient so they do not feel powerless to express their requirements during discussions. In some diverse groups and cultures, hierarchy and power are significantly valued. Another aspect to consider under the topic of relationship issues is gender and the way in which it is perceived within various groups. Be mindful when initially meeting with the patient of any gender differences that might cause unease. If you have any concerns, check with the patient if they have any specific preferences.

Experience

Your experience will improve by regular engagement with patients from diverse groups, and this will reduce any levels of anxiety that the nurse may experience. Prior to any meeting, you should prepare yourself by collecting as much information as possible about the patient and the purpose of the discussion. If there is the possibility of causing the patient distress, such as breaking bad news or the need to pose challenging questions, this should be done in a way that conveys sensitivity, respect and compassion. Communication is a two-way process, as highlighted in this chapter; as well as listening, patients will expect you to answer their questions. As a nurse, remember that you need to work within your capabilities and recognise your limitations, and if you have any doubts ask for help. As you will now appreciate from your reading of this section, there are a number of communication barriers that need consideration prior to and during communication with diverse groups.

Chapter summary

After reading this chapter, you should now have a good understanding of the importance of effective communication to improve health literacy in diverse groups. The vulnerability of such groups makes them more susceptible to less than adequate healthcare provision and poorer access. Health literacy remains a vast field of study, largely due to the recognition that patient and service user limitations in this area will impact negatively on health outcomes and life span. With the advent of an increasingly diverse group population and advances in healthcare, it is vital that we, as health professionals, continue to address the issues involving communication and health literacy. This will in turn narrow the gap and facilitate better access to services. Nurses must continually develop and maintain their communication skills to encompass all areas of verbal and non-verbal communication. This will provide quality individualised person-centred care that is both relevant and applicable to the diverse groups living in today's society.

Activities: brief outline answers

Activity 3.1   Reflection (p48)

Simon may well be feeling very scared, possibly stressed, as he is not in his normal environment and he is with staff who are not familiar to him. Added to this is the physiological symptom of pain, which is likely to cause increased anxiety and fear of what will happen. It is important that the way in which Simon is expressing himself, verbally and non-verbally, is taken into account. This may be more pronounced in persons with a learning disability (Chambers, 2003). There is a possibility that Simon might identify and interact better with Michael as he is a male nurse. Information will need to be obtained from as many sources as possible. This will enable staff to build a picture of Simon's usual behaviour; however, in the case study, it would appear that information is limited. Therefore, Kamala, Michael and Janet need to think of appropriate ways in which to engage with Simon. Aspects such as the tone of voice, body proximity, touch, language and the use of friendly words that Simon will understand can be helpful. Contact with a family member, friend or significant other will also alleviate fear and bring some normalisation to the situation for Simon, if contact is possible and appropriate. If available, the learning disability liaison nurse can provide expert advice. This role has been proven to have achieved positive outcomes for persons with learning disabilities admitted to hospital (Tuffrey-Wijne et al., 2013). While Michael has personal experience of learning disability, this is a work environment, and he might be feeling that as a student, he is there to learn rather than to share his knowledge. It is recommended that he should speak with Kamala and offer some suggestions. Michael might also wish to tell Kamala of his brother's condition if he feels comfortable enough to do so.

Activity 3.2   Communication and decision-making (p49)

In this scenario, Selina could be anxious and frightened due to her condition, and this will be increased by her mother's apparent refusal to accept the situation. It is likely that she might be feeling ill at ease despite having met Lucia previously. Schooling and social environment will impact upon Selina's understanding; however, at this age, it is likely that she will be asking questions, and Lucia must work to engage her in the discussion to ascertain her thoughts and feelings (Bach and Grant, 2015). The use of graphic materials will help to aid Selina's knowledge and promote participation. At this age, it is likely that Selina may be heavily influenced by her mother's behaviour. Therefore, in order to achieve a positive outcome to the meeting, it will be necessary to develop a productive relationship with Selina's mother. It will then be possible to explore her lack of acceptance and the reasons for this. Lucia will need to convey respect for the cultural background and appreciate the strongly held beliefs the mother might have. One way of approaching this is to ask the mother for more information about her health beliefs. The use of various communication techniques, such as allowing both Selina and her mother the opportunity to speak without interruption and not using jargon, will assist in reducing barriers. Lucia will also need to identify whether there are any illiteracy problems that are hindering the understanding of Selina or her mother. This will also demonstrate that Lucia is a collaborative partner in healthcare to work with, not against. Contact with other health professionals, such as the general practitioner (GP) and the consultant in charge of Selina's case, as well as the school, will be other sources of relevant information. As Selina is showing the physical symptom of tiredness, this will also require investigation as the diabetes might not be well controlled. If Lucia has any concerns about the vulnerability of Selina in the current situation, a safeguarding referral might be appropriate (HM Government, 2015). Safeguarding is about the right of individuals to be safe from harm; in relation to children, one of the key areas is the prevention of impairment of children's health or development. The NMC (2015) makes clear that we all have a role to play in safeguarding vulnerable adults and children in society. This would have to be discussed with Selina's parents so that they are fully informed and understand the reasons for this course of action, if deemed necessary.

Activity 3.4   Reflection and critical thinking (p54)

It is apparent from the scenario that Lazarus possesses some mental health literacy skills in terms of the continued treatment of his condition. There is significant relevance attached to the level of engagement and understanding of an individual's health condition. It is important to work with Lazarus by inviting him to a meeting to find out how much he does know about his schizophrenia and the treatment he is receiving. As mentioned earlier in the chapter, self-awareness is a key factor during collaboration with patients and service users. Recognition of how we, as healthcare professionals, present ourselves to others can have the potential to adversely affect the therapeutic relationship. The presence of Imran as an advocate is a necessary advantage, ensuring that Lazarus's autonomy is protected, and also as an intermediary if required. During the meeting, the language used and the information provided must be appropriate and acceptable to Lazarus, otherwise there will be no beneficial outcome. There may be a number of reasons why Lazarus has minimal health literacy skills; as identified in this chapter, these could range from poor literacy skills to ethnicity and gender. However, it could be the case that Lazarus has no motivation to engage with healthcare services. Alternatively, he may not want to inform his mother of the reason for the blood sample, or it might be that he has other support networks with whom he feels more comfortable discussing aspects of his health. It should be remembered that in terms of healthcare communication, not all individuals wish to have in-depth detail about their condition. As nurses, we need to recognise and gauge the patient or service user's requirements, and information should be tailored accordingly. The concern expressed by Lazarus's mother is to be expected; however, as an adult with full mental capacity, he is not compelled to talk to anyone about his health status unless he chooses to do so. It may be necessary for a member of the healthcare team to speak with Lazarus's mother to explain the relevance of privacy and confidentiality in terms of the disclosure of information that has not been consented to. The fact that Lazarus is willing to attend appointments is a positive factor in the management of his ongoing treatment.

Activity 3.7   Communication and reflection (p61)

From this scenario, it may be surmised that in the first context, the patient could be confused, frightened or in pain. In the second, it could be that the patient is comfortable and willing to be turned and is using her facial expression to communicate this to the nurse. It takes practice and experience to accurately interpret non-verbal communication, but it is a necessary skill that can be developed. We can conclude that in terms of non-verbal communication, facial expression is linked to certain emotions and is a powerful tool with which to communicate with others.

Further reading

Hart, P.L. and Moreno, N. (2016) Nurses' perceptions of their cultural competence in caring for diverse patient populations. *Online Journal of Cultural Competence in Nursing and Healthcare*, 6(1): 121–37. Available at: www.ojccnh.org/pdf/v6n1a10.pdf (accessed 7 April 2018).

The authors explore the perceived level of cultural competence skill held by nurses when caring for diverse patient populations. Their findings show that improvements are needed in terms of the provision of formal and continuing education.

Lamb, V. and Joels, C. (2014) Improving access to health care for homeless people. *Nursing Standard*, 29(6): 45–51.

This article provides an informed account of how homelessness is linked to social and health inequalities, and includes a practice case study.

NHS Improvement (2018) *The Learning Disability Improvement Standards for NHS Trusts.* Available at: https://improvement.nhs.uk/resources/learning-disability-improvement-standards-nhs-trusts/ (accessed 2 December 2018).

This document, produced by NHS Improvement, contains guidance on the standards of care to be delivered by all NHS trusts when patients with a learning disability, autism or both are admitted.

Nutbeam, D. (2008) The evolving concept of health literacy. *Social Science & Medicine*, 67: 2072–8.

This article debates the view of health literacy as a clinical risk or a personal asset, and provides the reader with a model for both to provoke further exploration of this concept.

Tuffrey-Wijne, I., Giatras, N., Goulding, L., Abraham, E., Fenwick, L., Edwards, C., et al. (2013) *Identifying the Factors Affecting the Implementation of Strategies to Promote a Safer Environment for Patients with Learning Disabilities in NHS Hospitals: A Mixed Methods Study.* Available at: www.journalslibrary.nihr.ac.uk/hsdr/hsdr01130/#/abstract (accessed 29 April 2018).

This is a study that looked into factors related to the promotion or compromise of a safe environment in NHS hospitals for patients with learning disabilities.

World Health Organization (WHO) (2013) *Health Literacy: The Solid Facts.* Available at: www.euro.who.int/__data/assets/pdf_file/0008/190655/e96854.pdf (accessed 28 April 2018).

An informative document that contains evidence in support of the need for a 'whole of society' approach to this concept.

Useful websites

Watch the following video, which explains the concept of paralanguage: **www.youtube.com/watch?v=FMoLkyrfp6o**

Cultural Diversity Network

www.culturaldiversitynetwork.co.uk

A global network that is concerned with culture and diversity and their relevance within the health of society and its economic development, as well as the promotion of cultural diversity.

Friends, Family and Travellers

www.gypsy-traveller.org/about-us

A national charity that works on behalf of all gypsy, Roma and traveller communities to ensure equity and justice by the provision of a wide range of services, advice and informative publications.

Health Literacy

www.healthliteracy.org

An American website that provides podcasts and information related to health literacy.

Health Literacy Out Loud

www.healthliteracyoutloud.com

An American website that contains useful podcasts and resources on a range of aspects focused upon health literacy.

Health Literacy Place

www.healthliteracyplace.org.uk

A Scottish-based resource website that provides information on aspects related to health literacy.

Mencap

www.mencap.org.uk

An organisation that is committed to raising awareness about all issues concerned with learning disability.

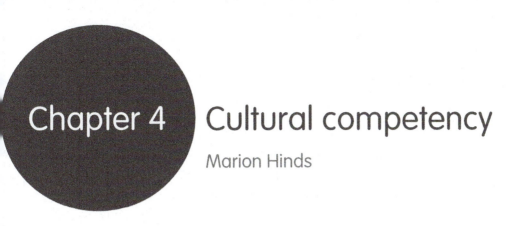

Chapter 4 Cultural competency

Marion Hinds

Chapter aims

After reading this chapter, you will be able to:

- define and explain the key terms 'culture', 'competence' and 'cultural competence';
- understand the relevant theory supporting the concepts of culture, competence and cultural competency, and their application to healthcare practice;
- understand the need for nurses to be culturally competent in healthcare settings; and
- apply knowledge and understanding to a range of work-based scenarios exploring cultural competence among patients, clients and service users.

Introduction

> ## Case study: Nurse who force-fed her baby
>
> In 2011, a Ghanaian nurse was found guilty of causing or allowing the death of her 10-month-old baby by force-feeding her liquidised food from small spouted china jugs over a number of months (Guardian Press Association, 2011). Force-feeding involved placing the spout into the child's mouth, effectively preventing her being able to close her mouth if she did not want any more food. The post-mortem examination concluded that pneumonia caused by foods, including meat and cereals, present in her lungs was the cause of death. The mother was described as being obsessed by her baby's weight and used this method of feeding when weaning her. She admitted that her baby often vomited after feeding but that she did not worry because her other children had done the same. It was claimed that the defendant had previously been warned by doctors and social workers about the dangers of this practice but ignored the advice (Guardian Press Association, 2011). She stated during the trial that this type of feeding was widely used and the way she and her siblings were fed by her mother in Ghana, and that she had done nothing to hurt her child. During the court proceedings, it was acknowledged that a death of this type, although rare, was a potential outcome of force-feeding. The prosecution stated, 'The mother, she is a nurse, and that involves a degree of extra insight. An ordinary mother would think twice or more before using a jug to pour food into the mouth of a child' (Guardian Press Association, 2011). The Chair of the Safeguarding Children Board confirmed that steps were being taken to provide better information nationally about this practice. The mother was subsequently convicted and sentenced to three years' imprisonment (Guardian Press Association, 2011). Her name was also permanently removed from the NMC register as her fitness to practise was found to be impaired by the nature of this conviction (NMC, 2012).

Culture is complex, as you may now appreciate after reading through the case study above and the previous chapters in this book. Culture is made up of many elements; some are clear to see, while others are not. The concept is generally viewed as shared notions, such as values, practices, beliefs and traditions, that are held by group members who identify as the same culture. These characteristics are in many cases strongly held, and are often passed on through generations, and can therefore be deeply rooted.

This purpose of this chapter is to explore the origin of cultural competency, the key terms 'culture', 'competence' and 'cultural competency', and the identification of two cultural competence theories and other key terminologies. The chapter will also examine a nursing model and its application in order to develop a holistic plan of care that will incorporate a patient's cultural identity. Discussion in this chapter will include the importance of knowledge, skill and attitude as essential traits that are required by all nurses in order to practise in an effective and safe manner. Key documents that focus upon competence will also be highlighted to demonstrate how they provide a bench-mark by which to measure the quality of care outcomes. A variety of activities and scenarios will guide you to link theory to practice and further develop an understanding of your own cultural competency.

Returning to the case study of the mother who force-fed her baby, it can be seen that one's culture encompasses both health and illness and can strongly influence areas of an individual's life. This includes aspects such as the timing when medical assistance is sought when unwell (Giger and Davidhizar, 2002) and the level of engagement that your patient will maintain in terms of recommended treatment regimes. Certain actions may be taken by the individual that are seen to be the 'right way of doing things', despite the possibility of causing harm. The case study highlights specific areas of consideration that add to the challenges when understanding the practices of people from different cultures. Three areas are worth discussion in relation to the case study:

1. *Mother's culture.* As already highlighted, culture is complex, and the mother will have been strongly influenced by her upbringing and the commonly held beliefs and values of her background. In the case study, it is evident that the mother was following traditional feeding practices that were carried on through generations in her family. The strength of these beliefs was demonstrated by evidence in court documents that showed she had been advised against the practice of force-feeding her baby by health and social professionals. What must also be taken into account is that in her experience, she had fed her older children in the same way and came to the conclusion that as no harm had come to them, there was nothing untoward with continuing with the practice. When conflict or discord occurs between people who hold differing cultural 'values, beliefs, assumptions and expectations of care', a culture or cultural clash is said to exist (Srivastava, 2003, p35). This clearly demonstrates the strong influence of one's cultural background.

2. *Professional nursing culture.* From a professional perspective, the mother was a registered nurse, and this would imply that she possessed a specific level of knowledge and skill in terms of health and illness. As a nurse, you are accountable in practice to ensure patient safety and that no harm comes to those in your care (NMC, 2015). A fundamental part of this is by the use of evidence-based interventions. The fact that the individual carried out this practice in her role as a mother does not condone her actions – hence the criminal charges laid against her. This is a challenging point of contention as the mother did not perceive herself as inflicting deliberate harm on her child.

3. *British culture.* In Western society, the biomedical model of healthcare is the most dominant. Its basis lies in the scientific and biological factors of illness and disease (Giddens and Sutton, 2017). Treatment is based upon interventions such as medication and surgical procedures by doctors and other qualified professionals.

However, the recent growth in alternative medicine, such as homeopathy, as another way to treat illness from a holistic perspective is becoming increasingly popular. People are now seeking other ways in which to treat sickness and disease. The practice of force-feeding, as seen in the case study, is a common and long-held tradition in some cultures as a way to ensure that a child will remain healthy and well-fed. However, in Western culture, this would not be seen as acceptable treatment of a child and would be viewed in terms of an act of cruelty.

It is easy to see from these three aspects of culture in relation to the case study that the concept is multifaceted and complex. The increasingly diverse nature of the population and various cultures (discussed in previous chapters) within modern Britain means that nurses are now, more than ever, likely to care for patients who have differing belief systems and concepts of health from their own. It is therefore important that an understanding of the components that lead to the development of cultural competence are a necessary prerequisite to the delivery of appropriate, effective and holistic nursing care (Henderson et al., 2018; O'Connell et al., 2007). It is impossible for you, as a student, to have knowledge of every culture or cultural identity. However, there is the need for nurses to be open and receptive to the development of their own individual cultural skill set (O'Hagan, 2001). In addition, as a nurse, you must also recognise and accept that your own beliefs, values and culture can – and will – influence all your healthcare encounters. This calls for the skill of self-awareness, which is discussed in the previous chapter.

In your role as a student nurse, it is worth remembering that even though culture can be a shared concept, it also tends to be unique to the individual (DeWilde and Burton, 2017). Just because two people share the same culture does not mean that they hold the same health beliefs and perform the same practices. Finally, remember that you are bound by the NMC code of conduct (NMC, 2015) and have a duty of care and candour to those in your care. You are required to take appropriate action should you witness any unlawful practices.

The previous chapters in this book have provided definitions of culture; however, the following definition offers a unique way in which to think about the term:

> *A term that applies to any group of people where there are common values and ways of thinking and acting that differ from those of another group.*

> (Srivastava, 2003, p15)

Another term commonly used is subculture, which is a component of culture. Subcultures exist within the mainstream or dominant culture. According to Giddens and Sutton (2017), a subculture is 'any segment of the population which is distinguishable from the wider society by its cultural pattern' (p1017). Examples of subcultures are:

- *religious* (e.g. Seventh-Day Adventists, Baptists, Mormons);
- *social/lifestyle* (e.g. LGBTQ, hip-hop music, naturists, online gamers); and
- *age* (e.g. elderly, youth culture).

After reading this section and Chapter 1, you should have a better understanding of the concept of culture and its relevance in nursing. Activity 4.1 asks you to reflect on your own culture and to list some of the specific characteristics that make it unique.

Activity 4.1 Reflection

In your own words, describe what you understand by the terms 'culture', 'competence' and 'cultural competency'.

What cultural background or identity would you describe yourself as?

List some of the specific characteristics of your cultural background or identity.

Download and read the following article, which discusses ways in which to achieve patient-centred care and develop the skills that will equip you in the development of cultural competence:

Campinha-Bacote, J. (2011) *Delivering Patient-Centred Care in the Midst of a Cultural Conflict: The Role of Cultural Competence.* Available at: http://ojin.nursingworld.org/MainMenuCategories/ANAMarketplace/ANAPeriodicals/OJIN/TableofContents/Vol-16-2011/No2-May-2011/Delivering-Patient-Centered-Care-in-the-Midst-of-a-Cultural-Conflict.html (accessed 13 August 2018).

An outline answer is provided at the end of the chapter.

Having read about culture in the previous section, we now move on to explore the meaning of competence, competency and cultural competency, in addition to some key supporting theory.

Competence, competency and cultural competency

Becoming a registered nurse means that you are a professional, and therefore accountable for your practice; part of professionalism is the achievement of competence (NMC, 2017). The NMC code makes clear that nurses must maintain competence in order to practise as a registered nurse, and performance that falls below this standard will be subject to scrutiny. You must also 'recognise and work within the limits of your competence' (NMC, 2015, p11). Essentially, nursing competence should be viewed as a holistic notion that encompasses not only the requisite knowledge and skills, but an appropriate attitude that conveys the unique art and skill of caring as a nurse. Competence is a generic quality and refers to an individual's capacity to perform job responsibilities, while competency is the actual performance or ability to do something in a specific situation (McConnell, 2001). Competent is defined as 'having the necessary ability, knowledge or skill to do something successfully' (Lexico, 2019b).

It is important to define competence because, as a student nurse, successful achievement will allow you to register with the Nursing and Midwifery Council. It also establishes the role of the nurse from a professional viewpoint (Fukada, 2018). Competence is gained through experience and learning, and it is described as a characteristic of behaviour (Fukada, 2018). As a student, you may already be familiar with a definition of competence or competency as during your practice placements you are required to achieve a certain level of performance for successful progression. Throughout your training, you will complete mandatory training sessions, such as manual handling and lifting and basic life support. These are necessary to ensure that when you attend practice placements, you are sufficiently prepared with the underpinning knowledge and understanding to perform specific tasks and skills. This does not mean that you are competent; you will need further practice in the clinical setting in order to develop.

The Royal College of Nursing Principles of Nursing Practice provide succinct commentary on what everyone, patients and nurses themselves, can expect from nursing practice (RCN, 2010). Principle F specifically addresses that healthcare professionals have 'up to date knowledge and skills, and use these with intelligence, insight and understanding in line with the needs of each individual in their care'. Therefore, as a nurse, you must continue to engage with ongoing continuing professional development. A key issue with competence is that it can be dependent upon the particular situation or circumstance. Therefore, nurses are expected to use and adapt their underlying knowledge and skills to the environment in which they find themselves. In consideration of the above, the development and maintenance of competence and competency can be problematic if not practised on a regular basis so that you become familiar with the subject matter and skills involved (McConnell, 2001). That is why, in your role as a nurse, it is necessary, in line with the NMC code of practice (NMC, 2015), that you keep your knowledge and skills up to date.

However, your attitude is just as important as your knowledge and skills, and during your clinical placements you will be aware that you are assessed in the three domains of knowledge, skill and attitude. One of the findings from the Francis Report on the failings of Mid Staffordshire Trust was that some staff attitudes were described as 'leaving much to be desired' (Department of Health, 2013).

The Compassion in Practice document cites competence as one of the 6 Cs, and states that 'all those in caring roles must have the ability to understand an individual's health and social needs and the expertise, clinical and technical knowledge to deliver effective care and treatments based on research and evidence' (NHS England, 2012). There are various definitions of cultural competence, and it is universally acknowledged as an essential skill for healthcare professionals, as well as a prerequisite for positive health outcomes. Ongoing debate continues as to how to best define the term, with Bettancourt et al. (2013) citing that it is a 'broad construct' (p293), and this is possibly the challenge in finding a fixed interpretation. The authors continue that it is:

understanding the importance of social and cultural influences on patients' health beliefs and behaviours; considering how these factors interact at multiple levels of the health care delivery system (e.g., at the level of structural processes of care or clinical decision making), and finally devising interventions that take these issues into account to assure quality health care delivery to diverse patient populations.

(p297)

The origin of cultural competence study began with Madeleine Leininger (1925–2012), who advocated the need for culturally competent nursing care due to the apparent lack of awareness of the need to recognise the importance of culture in care. Imbedded in this was the need for nurses to be able to function effectively when caring for people from different cultures in her prediction of an increasingly multicultural world. Leininger (1995) described the concept of transcultural nursing as:

a formal area of study and practice focused on comparative holistic cultural care, health and illness patterns of individuals and groups with respect to differences and similarities in cultural values, beliefs and practices with the goal to provide culturally congruent, sensitive, and competent nursing care to people of diverse cultures.

(p4)

Another well-known leader in the field of cultural competence is Josepha Campinha-Bacote (2002), who described it as an ongoing process in which healthcare providers continually try to work in an effective manner within the cultural context of their clients. Simply put, it is the development of underpinning knowledge, skills and attitudes in order to provide effective care to people from different cultural backgrounds. The field of transcultural nursing is described by Maria Jirwe, Kate Gerrish and Azita Emami as that which helps nurses to become culturally competent (Jirwe et al., 2006).

Other well-known authors of cultural competence theory are Irena Papadopoulos, Mary Tilki and Gina Taylor, who together produced a model for the development of cultural competence (Papadopoulos et al., 1998). Their definition sees it as providing effective healthcare to others while taking into consideration their cultural beliefs, behaviours and needs. The term 'cultural competence' is seen as the end goal in the development of key skills such as cultural awareness, cultural sensitivity and cultural knowledge, which are well noted characteristics of the theory. Other facets, such as cultural desire and cultural encounter, have been included to provide a more comprehensive picture of the entire process from beginning to end. These terms are discussed later in this chapter in the section on cultural competence models.

Henderson et al. (2018, p590) concluded in their study on cultural competence in community healthcare that it has a positive effect on patients, related to satisfaction of care, quality, effective interactions and improved health outcomes.

Your reading so far has introduced you to the meanings of competence, competency and cultural competency, and how these underpin nursing practice. Activity 4.2 asks you to consider your own experience, preparation and knowledge in the care of patients from different cultural groups.

> ## Activity 4.2   Critical thinking and reflection
>
> Think about your last placement. How much information or preparation were you given by your practice assessor or any other healthcare professional about the different cultural groups/patients that you might meet?
>
> If you did not receive any information or preparation, what do you think you need to know and be prepared for when caring for different cultural groups/patients?
>
> Discuss these with your practice assessor next time you are in placement and consider ways to address any challenges in the delivery of patient-centred care to different cultural groups/patients.
>
> Choose a cultural group that you would like to find out more about. Take time out to research and make notes on the group you have chosen.
>
> *There is an outline answer at the end of the chapter.*

After reading the previous section, you should now have an appreciation of why it is important in nursing practice to understand competence and its application in the care of patients from various cultures.

The next section will begin with a discussion of the Roper–Logan–Tierney model of nursing, which is the most frequently used in the United Kingdom (UK) (Roper et al., 2002). This will demonstrate the relevance of a nursing model before learning about cultural competency models later in this chapter.

Nursing models

A key purpose of a nursing model is to collect information so the nurse can perform a holistic patient assessment in a structured manner. You will then be able to develop an individualised plan that will facilitate and promote the continuity of care. By using a model, you can find out and review pertinent information that can be used to ascertain the patient's current and previous health status and identify nursing problems. From a professional perspective, according to Barrett et al. (2019), a model provides a picture of what nursing is and gives 'direction to the nurse about patients and their needs, they define nursing roles' (p43). The specific model that we shall focus upon in this section is the Roper–Logan–Tierney model (Roper et al., 2002), which is founded upon the

12 activities of living (AL). All activities relate to an individual's day-to-day functioning and will be relevant. However, dependent upon the patient circumstances, not all will be applicable at the time of the patient interaction (you will see why in Activity 4.7). These activities are:

- maintaining a safe environment;
- communication;
- breathing;
- eating and drinking;
- elimination;
- personal cleansing and dressing;
- controlling body temperature;
- mobilising;
- working and playing;
- expressing sexuality;
- sleeping; and
- dying.

However, while these are applicable to every day, an individual's cultural needs may not be immediately obvious when using the model. It is therefore possible for you, as a student, to carry out an assessment using the AL model without being alerted to any particular cultural values and preferences. This can happen between an inexperienced nurse and a patient who does not wish to divulge any cultural beliefs or values, particularly if they are not immediately apparent.

As a nurse, you will be aware that the first part of the nursing process is the patient assessment. This is key in order for you to collect valid and relevant information from your patient, and this can take time, dependent upon the type of admission. For example, in an emergency situation, there may not be much information that you can gather if the patient is unconscious. In that case, you would need to obtain information from other sources. Purnell (2016) stipulates that culturally congruent care will be achieved by gathering as much information as possible about the patient's culture during the assessment process. Culturally congruent care is that which 'incorporates key values and beliefs of the client in a given situation' (Srivastava, 2003, p56). You will need to pay attention to the style of verbal and non-verbal communication employed by the patient, as well as your use of language that can be understood. This will help to build rapport and promote an environment in which the patient is comfortable enough to express their needs without fear of negative judgement or being misunderstood. The patient assessment will allow you to identify and prioritise the patient problem. Remember that the patient assessment stage is an ongoing and continuous process, and not a one-off task, which is why Roper et al. (2002) prefer the term 'assessing' rather than 'assessment' (p124).

The following scenario will help you to apply the Roper–Logan–Tierney activities of living model to a specific patient scenario involving Sheila, a Jehovah's Witness.

> ## Scenario: Jehovah's Witness patient
>
> Imagine you are admitting 55-year-old Sheila to the overnight stay surgical ward for a planned routine procedure. This is her first time being admitted to hospital, and Sheila did not want any treatment, but her symptoms of chronic tiredness and anaemia meant that she was recommended for further examination. During the admission process, when you ask if she has any religious or spiritual beliefs, she tells you that she is a practising Jehovah's Witness. Sheila admits that she is nervous about the operation, and also that she was informed by the consultant that there was a possibility she might need a blood transfusion. As this is against her beliefs, she is adamant that she does not want this type of intervention. Sheila wants reassurance from you that she will not be given a blood transfusion.

Activity 4.3 will now help you to think more critically and reflect upon how you can apply the activities of living (AL) model to assess Sheila's cultural needs.

Activity 4.3   Critical thinking and reflection

Read Chapter 2, 'The model of living', in Roper et al. (2002), which will provide you with the underpinning knowledge and understanding in relation to the activities of living (AL). Consider what further information you might need to obtain from Sheila to provide a culturally appropriate assessment that takes into account her specific needs.

An outline answer can be found at the end of the chapter.

After completing Activity 4.3, you should have a much clearer idea of how to use the AL framework to assess your patients' cultural needs. We will now move on to read about two cultural competence models of care, their key purpose being to ensure that patients are seen for who they are and their uniqueness. Care will then be delivered in a culturally appropriate, sensitive and holistic manner.

Cultural competence models

The next section will outline three cultural competence models: (1) Campinha-Bacote's process of cultural competence in the delivery of healthcare services (Campinha-Bacote, 2002); (2) Papadopoulos, Tilki and Taylor's (PTT) model of developing cultural competence (Papadopoulos et al., 1998); and (3) the Papadopoulos culturally competent compassion model (Papadopoulos, 2014). You will need to understand how these interconnect with each other and form a foundation for cultural competency and culturally competent care.

While you are reading this section, think about how skilled you consider yourself to be in each area and how you could demonstrate these skills in practical and theoretical terms.

Campinha-Bacote's process of cultural competence in the delivery of healthcare services (Campinha-Bacote, 2002)

The author cites five distinct areas that make up the basis of this body of study, which are described here.

Cultural awareness

This is the conscious recognition that other cultures exist and an appreciation that not everyone comes from the same cultural background. During interactions with others from a different culture, nurses should be mindful of their own feeling and any biases they might hold. This calls for an honest evaluation of oneself, which may be difficult for some. It is a key aspect, as mentioned earlier in this chapter, as our values and beliefs will influence the care we deliver. You will need to begin by using self-reflection to answer questions such as: Are there individual patients or groups of patients that I see or treat differently from others, and why is this? In order to have awareness, as a nurse, you must be receptive and open to new or different ways of learning about others. In addition, those in your care may have very little in common with you, and vice versa, which may be challenging. Remember that by demonstrating a level of mindfulness of cultural differences, you will enable positive change to take place between those involved in the interaction.

Cultural knowledge

This is a significant factor in the development of cultural competence. Your ability to use knowledge of different beliefs, practices and values is necessary to aid decision-making in terms of providing safe and appropriate patient care. The nurse's level of knowledge will depend upon previous, current and ongoing experience of cultural interactions with different groups. We can therefore acknowledge that this is a continuous process (Campinha-Bacote, 2002; Papadopoulos et al., 1998). Nurses should actively engage in seeking factual information and participate in training opportunities so as to understand various patient beliefs about health and illness. A solid knowledge base underpinned with practice learning can prevent misconceptions and stereotyping based upon preconceived ideologies.

Cultural skill

The requirement to obtain factual information that will form the basis of a comprehensive patient assessment is necessary for the treatment of all patients. With patients from different cultures, this is even more important, as there may be serious implications to the continuity of care. A lack of appreciation and recognition of culturally relevant information can impact areas such as non-engagement with the assessment and adherence to recommended treatment. Cultural skill includes not only obtaining information, but being able to process and utilise this for the good of the patient. Part of cultural skill is finding out the patient's perception of their illness and the LEARN mnemonic (Berlin and Fowkes, 1983) offers a way in which to facilitate this exchange. The more skill gained in this area, the more comfortable the nurse will become in the art of cultural assessment.

Cultural encounter

This involves the way in which the nurse directly engages with the patient in the exchange of information and will incorporate a number of variables. Consideration of the level of health literacy (see Chapter 3) is a starting point and will have implications in terms of the success of the encounter. There is likely to be communication differences, and these need to be acknowledged and ways found to address these in a manner that is acceptable to the patient (e.g. the use of translator services). With reference to body language and interaction, in some cultures, particularly African cultures, the left hand is perceived as inferior to the right, and there are instances when children are discouraged from using the left hand to write (Adekoya and Ogunola, 2015). Therefore, if an older patient from this culture were to be assessed by a nurse who was left-handed, this could prove to be problematic (e.g. an introductory handshake using the left hand would be considered disrespectful). Cultural encounter also includes the setting where this process takes place, and as far as possible aspects of privacy should be taken into account by using a setting with minimal disruptions. As identified at the start of this chapter, in the case study, a cultural clash is a factor that should not be overlooked. To prevent this, sensitivity and respect must be conveyed to the patient, as well as the recognition of the acceptance of another. The value that can be gained by holding conversations with patients from different cultural groups should not be underestimated, offering you, as a nurse, the opportunity to gain valuable experiential learning in practice. Further information about communication and environment can be found in Chapter 3.

Cultural desire

The concept of cultural desire implies that it is something that you want to do and that a degree of motivation will be required in order achieve this skill. As a student, you may or may not have come across patients with differing cultural backgrounds to yours. As nurses, we must take the time to consider and learn about the health and illness beliefs of those from different cultural backgrounds in order to provide holistic individualised care.

The next model we will look at is Papadopoulos, Tilki and Taylor's model of developing cultural competence. You will notice that there is some replication of section headings in this and the previous model.

Papadopoulos, Tilki and Taylor's (PTT) model of developing cultural competence (Papadopoulos et al., 1998)

This model consists of four main concepts that lead to cultural competence.

Cultural awareness

Consider the influence of stereotyping individuals and how that will influence your behaviour towards patients from different cultures. This type of behaviour stems from a lack of awareness of the difference of others.

Cultural knowledge

In this area, the authors recognise the impact of knowledge, and at a fundamental level question the production and origin of this specific knowledge (Papadopoulos, 2006, p13). This is an important consideration in the quest for cultural competence, as without knowledge of culture one cannot have a basis upon which to develop. The subject of health inequality is a key component of this model in relation to exploring why this still occurs, and the authors concede that further research is required in this area.

Cultural sensitivity

During interactions with different cultures we must take care to recognise the impact that these differences might have, so as not to cause offence. Sensitivity is about the way in which we perceive patients from different cultures who are in our care. As nurses, we also need to reflect on how patients see us. If we are unable to work with our patients in an environment of trust and respect, there will be a breakdown in the nurse–patient relationship, which will lead to a negative outcome. In order to develop effective relationships with our patients, good communication and collaborative practice are required. If you are unsure about any aspect of your patient's culture, beliefs or preferences, as highlighted in the scenario about Esme (page 86) and discussed in Chapter 3, you must ask for help from your practice assessor or another member of staff.

Cultural competence

This is the accomplishment of the above stages, which then culminate in competence. A noticeable element of competence is the ability of the nurse to address and challenge any negative behaviour, such as discrimination, inequalities and prejudice. This is, however, an ongoing process of learning and development.

Papadopoulos's culturally competent compassion model (Papadopoulos, 2014)

The delivery of nursing care that shows compassion is of such significance that it is cited as one of the 6 Cs (NHS England, 2012), which are benchmarks for the provision of nursing care that demonstrates the values of dignity and respect to patients.

The art of compassion has been defined by Perez-Bret et al. (2016) as:

> *the sensitivity shown in order to understand another person's suffering, combined with a willingness to help and to promote the well-being of that person, in order to find a solution to their situation.*

(p605)

The authors also comment that 'Compassionate care can be shown with words, but also by a silent, caring and respectful attitude' (p603). Culturally competent compassion is defined by Papadopoulos and Pezella (2015) as:

> *the human quality of understanding the suffering of others and wanting to do something about it, using culturally appropriate and acceptable interventions, which take into consideration both the patients' and the carers' cultural backgrounds as well as the context in which care is given.*

(p2)

The model of culturally competent compassion consists of four constructs that, as you will see, are extensions of the subsections that make up the PTT model of developing cultural competence, which we have covered in the section above:

1. cultural awareness and compassion;
2. cultural knowledge and compassion;
3. cultural sensitivity and compassion; and
4. cultural competence and compassion.

The key aspect to this new model by Papadopoulos (2014) is the requirement for healthcare professionals to understand the concept and implications of cultural competence combined with the quality of compassion. The very nature of nursing means that without this, we cannot hope to practise effectively, nor see others and what they represent. A number of definitions have been provided above for the concept of compassion, and, as indicated by Papadopoulos (2014), it is a quality that is at the heart of clinical practice. Without compassion as a behavioural trait, care cannot be effective, nor humanely delivered, which without doubt is key in the delivery of culturally competent nursing care.

This section will have provided you with an understanding of the underpinning theory and application to practice of two of the key cultural competence frameworks.

There are other cultural competence models contained in nursing literature that you can research in your own time in order to widen your knowledge base in this subject area. The next section will continue by presenting an example framework that can be used in practice to reduce challenges in the delivery of culturally appropriate nursing care.

Challenges to the delivery of culturally appropriate care

From what you have read so far in this chapter, you may now appreciate that there are a number of challenges and potential barriers that can impede the delivery of culturally appropriate care. These may originate from a number of perspectives. A key one is the quality of interaction between the nurse and the patient, as identified by, but not limited to, the discussion on cultural encounter and cultural sensitivity. If there are difficulties, an avoidable breakdown will occur. Negative stereotyping and a lack of understanding towards an individual's cultural background by any health professional will ultimately lead to alienation and lack of engagement by the patient with healthcare services. By conscious consideration and implementation of the stages described in the models, you too can develop the skills to reduce the challenges so as to provide an appropriate level of cultural care. The LEARN model of cross-cultural encounters (Berlin and Fowkes, 1983) is a guideline of principles devised in recognition of the necessity for healthcare workers to productively engage with patients from different cultural backgrounds. It is based on a mnemonic as follows:

> *Listen with sympathy and understanding to the patient's perception of the problem.*
>
> *Explain your perceptions of the problem.*
>
> *Acknowledge and discuss the differences and similarities of those involved in the interaction.*
>
> *Recommend treatment based upon the patient's requirements.*
>
> *Negotiate agreement with the patient to facilitate co-operation.*

(p934)

By following this framework, the nurse can engage in a meaningful way with the patient to promote understanding and collaboration in order to positively address healthcare needs. By utilising LEARN, the authors surmise that the quality of the assessment should improve, by enabling the patient to express in their own unique way, and from their perspective, what concerns they might have.

Quality is a measurable outcome and is an indication of the effectiveness of nursing care. The following section will now look at some of the quality developments that influence the delivery of cultural care.

Quality and cultural care

The ability to deliver an appropriate level of care is of particular importance in this discussion on cultural competency as patient satisfaction and the subjective experience are key indicators of quality in the provision of NHS services. Everyone has their own idea of what quality means to them, and this will vary dependent upon a variety of things. The term 'quality' is usually seen as 'the standard of something as measured against things of a similar kind; the degree of excellence of something' (Lexico, 2019c). According to Glen (1998), the values that matter to us are a major influence in the delivery of 'high quality nursing care' (p38). As highlighted in the Francis Report (Department of Health, 2013), basic nursing care fell short of the standard expected, and to a certain extent this might explain why frequent instances of poor care and such variations existed.

High Quality Care for All by Lord Darzi (2008) stated that:

> *High quality care should be as safe and effective as possible, with patients treated with compassion, dignity and respect. As well as clinical quality and safety, quality means care that is personal to each individual.*

(p11)

The Nursing and Midwifery Council has recently published new standards of proficiency for registered nurses and midwives to reflect the changing role of nursing in the twenty-first century (NMC, 2018). There has long been the recognition that the role of the nurse is becoming more complex in line with the changing demographic and population make-up of the UK. As a nurse, the NMC (2018) makes clear that you are expected to deliver care to individuals of all ages from different backgrounds, cultures and beliefs. In addition, a legal obligation is imposed in the duty of care, as well as accountability for any actions in the delivery of that care to patients within your remit (NMC, 2018; RCN, 2010). Care must be patient-centred, compassionate, and address an individual's physical, spiritual and psychological needs, and these are linked to the concept of quality. Person-centred or individualised care is 'an approach where the person is at the centre of the decision making processes and the design of their care needs, their nursing care and treatment plan' (NMC, 2018, p35). The NICE quality standard 15 makes note in quality statement 4 that 'patients have opportunities to discuss their health beliefs, concerns and preferences to inform their individualised care' (NICE, 2012). So, as an example indicator of quality and patient-centred care, healthcare professionals should provide information that is accessed easily and understood by the patient. If not, this can lead to dissatisfaction, non-engagement and poor-quality care, as highlighted in Chapter 3. Another example could be that during the admission process, nurses are mindful to ask about the patient's cultural background and religious and spiritual needs. Quality care, as you will have understood from this section so far, includes safety. *Cultural safety* is healthcare that recognises the importance of collaboration with patients in an environment that fosters a therapeutic relationship, taking into account the recipient's cultural needs. You will be able to read more about the influence of religion when you read the scenario featuring Esme in Activity 4.5. Competent practice in your role as a nurse includes the necessary use of up-to-date evidence-based practice, which is another indicator of quality (NMC, 2015).

You will now be aware of the importance of quality as a key component in the delivery of cultural care. Complete Activity 4.4 as this will enable you to reflect on the 6 Cs and their application to patient-centred care.

Activity 4.4　Critical thinking and reflection

Read Baillie (2017). It will provide you with further information on the application of the 6 Cs as a foundation for patient-centred nursing care.

There is no answer at the end of the chapter as it is based upon your own understanding of the article's content.

After reading the information in this chapter so far, you need to consider what it is necessary for you to know about a patient's culture in order to provide the best possible care. According to O'Connell et al. (2007), 'if practitioners have culturally competent attitudes, knowledge, and skills, care can be improved for all patients' (p1062).

With a focus on culture, religion and spirituality, the next section will develop your knowledge and skills in relation to these themes.

Culture, religion and spirituality

Society today is filled with challenges in terms of equality in healthcare delivery to an ever-increasing multicultural society, some of whom are described as the most vulnerable. As a nurse, you are in a unique position to develop the knowledge, skills and attitudes to address some of these challenging issues. In accordance with the NMC code, you are to prioritise people; therefore, you need to examine your own values and beliefs about others so that you are able to function in an effective manner when caring for all patients (NMC, 2015, 1.3). Negative views, such as prejudice, cultural stereotyping and cultural bias, will hinder your ability to overcome cultural differences and build appropriate therapeutic relationships. A relationship that is therapeutic is two-way, enhances the patient experience by way of the nurse and patient working together, and involves empathy, genuineness and respect (Peplau, 1987).

There are close links between culture, religion and spirituality, and in many ways they appear intertwined. As nurses, we must take note of and respect a patient's right to practise and uphold their traditional religious beliefs, even if we do not agree with or hold any particular beliefs ourselves. The NMC (2018) makes clear that, as nurses, we must integrate spirituality into our nursing practice. However, according to Hordern (2016), this should not condone unlawful action nor serve as 'the approval or endorsement of any particular belief' (p590). Religion is described as a more formal and organised system of practice with recognised customary celebrations, and most importantly the worship of God (Santori, 2010). Alternatively, spirituality has no religious attachment, relates to the 'spirit or soul', and can be seen as a 'quest to understand the true meaning of life' (Santori, 2010, p15). Ledger and Bowler (2013) discuss the spiritual needs of mental health patients. They acknowledge that 'patient-centred holistic care' in mental health service provision must involve the recognition of spirituality as 'a key aspect' (p21). Religious and spiritual needs are most commonly considered when a patient is approaching the end of life as patients often find comfort in seeking meaning and peace in their lives. The NMC (2018) state that nurses should 'recognise and respond compassionately to the needs of those who are in the last few days and hours of life' (p7). The RCN guide on culture and spirituality provides some outline information for nurses on this subject (RCN, 2016b).

As healthcare professionals, we should also be mindful that patients will have varying levels of personal compliance in terms of their beliefs. For patients who hold strong religious views with strict adherence to certain rituals, there can be wide-ranging implications when they become ill and are admitted to hospital. This can involve issues such as the refusal of medical interventions, non-acceptance of pain relief, non-acceptance of the existence of mental health conditions, and aspects of end-of-life care. There are positive benefits to patient well-being when cultural, religious and spiritual needs are met by healthcare professionals (Rogers and Wattis, 2015; Timmins and Caldeira, 2017a).

You will now have developed an understanding of the importance of recognising the relevance of a patient's religious and spiritual needs. Read the following scenario about Esme, an elderly Jewish lady.

Scenario: Religion and food preference

Esme is a 78-year-old Jewish woman who is transferred to the ward. Shanique, a first-year student nurse, is allocated to care for her with the supervision of her practice assessor. It is lunchtime, and Shanique brings Esme her kosher meal, and being helpful proceeds to open the plastic covering. She is about to unwrap the cutlery when she notices that Esme has become very upset and tearful and refuses to eat the food. Esme will not explain why, and Shanique is confused and unsure of what to do. She leaves Esme to go to find her practice assessor for assistance.

Now read and complete Activity 4.5.

Activity 4.5   Reflection and critical thinking

After reading the scenario about Esme, answer the following questions:

- What do you think has occurred in this situation?
- How do you think Esme is feeling?
- Could Shanique have done anything differently?
- Imagine that you and your practice assessor are admitting Esme. What questions do you need to ask her in order to complete an assessment that will consider her religious and spiritual requirements?

There is a model answer to these questions at the end of the chapter.

After reading the previous section, you should now have a better idea of the importance of culture, religion and beliefs. A lack of awareness in relation to the possible issues that may occur will inadvertently cause offence to those in your care.

This section will consider a scenario in which the mother does not wish to vaccinate her child due to her religious beliefs.

Read the following scenario and answer the questions in Activity 4.6. You will then be able to consider the knowledge you have gained so far in terms of cultural competence.

Scenario: Baby vaccination

Imagine you are a first-year student nurse on placement in the community and are spending the day with the GP practice nurse, Nada. Bushra, a 25-year-old Muslim woman who has recently moved into the area, has brought her 3-year-old son, Jareem, to see the GP, Dr Oros, who originates from Romania. She is concerned about Jareem's recurrent cold and flu symptoms. Jareem is sitting on his mother's lap and is clingy towards her; he has a runny nose and a slight cough. This is the second time Dr Oros has seen Jareem in the past six days, and he has advised Bushra that due to the frequency of his symptoms over the past six months, he should be given the nasal flu vaccine; however, she has refused. The GP is frustrated by this situation, particularly due to the fact that he feels that Bushra lacks engagement with him during discussions. He calls Nada into the consulting room to meet Bushra in the hope that she might be able to persuade her to allow Jareem to be vaccinated. When you enter the consulting room with Nada, Bushra seems happy to see you both. Dr Oros

(Continued)

(Continued)

decides to leave the room. Nada starts with introductions and asks Bushra to explain what the problem is. Bushra becomes upset as she explains that her son is having frequent cold and flu symptoms and she does not know why. She also states that Dr Oros keeps pushing her to agree to the flu vaccine being given to Jareem, but she is not happy about this. Bushra says that she has heard that the medicine contains gelatine and it is against her religious beliefs to allow him to have anything containing pork. Nada explains to Bushra that she has previously spoken to a number of Muslim parents about the flu vaccine and is happy to provide her with more information. In your student experience so far, you have not had much interaction with people from a Muslim background and are confused by Bushra's decision not to protect her child against recurrent cold and flu symptoms.

Activity 4.6   Decision-making and leadership

After reading the above scenario, answer the following questions:

- What are the key issues for consideration in this scenario?
- What actions do you think Nada should take?
- As a student nurse, what questions might you ask Nada following the consultation with Bushra?

An outline answer can be found at the end of the chapter.

After reading the scenario and completing Activity 4.6, you will realise that cultural competence does not necessarily mean that the healthcare professional is an expert in all aspects of this field. However, the recognition that culture is a fundamental part of the nursing role and of the patients we meet is a well-intentioned starting point.

Chapter summary

Inevitably, during your practice, you will come across individuals from different cultures with values and beliefs that are unlike your own. Cultural skill awareness and the ongoing pursuit of cultural competence is a requirement for all healthcare professionals in order to address the needs of patients from different backgrounds. Competence needs to be demonstrated in meaningful ways through education and also exposure to practice so that skills can be improved. Communication and a desire to deliver quality care that is respectful and demonstrates dignity to those with different cultural needs and beliefs should be a common goal for all those involved in the delivery of nursing care. As a nurse, reflect on your clinical skill, knowledge and practice in terms of how you relate to and care for patients in a culturally appropriate manner. Take the opportunity to discuss cultural care with your practice assessor and others in the clinical environment. It is to our detriment, in today's society, if we fail to do so.

Activities: brief outline answers

Activity 4.1   Reflection (p73)

Culture, competence and cultural competency will be described in your own words, but you can find the definitions of these terms in this and previous chapters of this book.

As an example of a cultural background/identity: Alessa is 20 years of age and was born in the UK to Italian parents, who she lives with, as well as her two older siblings. She classifies herself as white British and has both a British and Italian passport. Alessa's upbringing was very strict; her parents are practising Catholics and the influence of religious observance is highly revered in her family. Her Italian grandparents also live in the family home, and when Alessa is not working she is very involved in caring for them in light of their declining health. The entire family is very close, and evening mealtimes are very important to her parents, who expect everyone to be around the table to spend time together.

Activity 4.2   Critical thinking and reflection (p76)

During the orientation period of your last placement, you may or may not have been given any information or preparation by your practice assessor about the needs of patients from different cultures. It is good practice to make a conscious effort in each clinical placement you attend to ask questions about the different cultures of patients admitted to the ward. You should then spend some time researching and making notes for your information. The Royal College of Nursing have produced a toolkit with information aimed at helping students to make the most of their practice placements (RCN, 2017a). The document states that an effective practice placement should support you to:

- *Recognise cultural variance and develop cultural competence.*
- *Develop confidence in delivering person-centred care.*

(p6)

The placement area should have guidelines that relate specifically to the most common cultural groups that you will encounter, so make sure that you read them. Reflect upon what action you will take when you initially care for a patient from a different culture and what questions you will need to ask in order to deliver culturally appropriate care. This could include:

- Consider setting an objective in your assessment document to address the development of cultural competency.
- Read the patient's medical and nursing notes and familiarise yourself with relevant information, such as language spoken, reason for admission, diagnosis and current health status.
- Before approaching the patient (you may be in the company of your practice assessor), ensure that you are clear as to what you are going to be doing with/to the patient (i.e. that you are working within your limitations).

- Introduce yourself and ask if they have a preferred name/title that they would like to be known as.
- Do not be afraid to ask the patient questions in an appropriate manner about their cultural background. As previously mentioned, most patients will not mind as long as you explain your reason for doing so.
- If the situation allows, find out as much information as you can about the patient's preferences, values, beliefs and traditions, particularly if they may have implications on the hospital stay. Do not forget to include significant others and family members.
- Document the information you obtain in the patient's notes and inform your practice assessor.
- Think about any possible challenges in the ward environment that may hinder the provision of cultural care to your patient.
- Afterwards, discuss the encounter with your practice assessor and reflect on the interaction.

Activity 4.3   Critical thinking and reflection (p78)

There are a number of aspects that will need to be considered during your assessment of Sheila under the activity of maintaining a safe environment in order to promote patient safety. Maintaining a safe environment is concerned with the internal and external environment, and harm can occur from many sources. Sheila has an increased level of anxiety about the surgical procedure, and therefore it is important to find out what her specific concerns are. Further information must be provided by nursing staff and the surgical team involved with Sheila's care to alleviate her worries. The team will need to be informed of her concerns as Sheila will require further review prior to surgery. Information leaflets can be provided for her to read in her own time, and you should advise her to ask if there is anything that she does not understand. Sheila's religion prohibits the use of blood, which stems from biblical beliefs. There are a number of biblical verses, such as Genesis 9:4 and Leviticus 17:10, that command followers to abstain from blood, which is seen to be a representation of life (Jehovah's Witnesses, 2018). It will be necessary for you to confirm with her if this includes blood derivatives such as fresh frozen plasma (FFP) and human albumin solution (HAS). There are other options, such as autotransfusion, which might be a more acceptable alternative. This process involves the removal and reintroduction of the patient's own blood into their circulatory system. It is important that Sheila has a fully informed understanding of her decision and that she is well within her rights to exercise her refusal. You could suggest that she speaks with a trusted elder or significant other in her congregation for further advice. As the admitting nurse, you must ensure that you clearly document the information collected and that this is relayed to the rest of the nursing team. When available, all relevant test results must be contained in the notes. You will also need to find out if Sheila has any other past medical history or if she is taking any regular medications, and document this information in her notes.

Activity 4.5   Reflection and critical thinking (p87)

Adequate nutritional intake is necessary for patient recovery and well-being. In some cultural groups, there are strict rules to be followed concerning dietary habits. Religion is usually the most common reason for food restrictions. Any deviation, unless for an exceptional reason, can be seen as a disregard for the fundamental belief principles of the specific group. Healthcare professionals should develop an awareness of common religious food habits to avoid causing offence and ask the patient if they are unsure. Religious observances are a way of life and exert a very strong influence in some cultural groups. As a student nurse caring for these individuals, you must appreciate the impact of religious beliefs and their importance in relation to care delivery (Mendes, 2015; Sartori, 2010). This includes the need to demonstrate dignity and respect by treating them as individuals and tailoring care in conjunction with this. Jewish traditions concerning dietary habits are that all meals must be prepared and served by observance of kashrut, which is kosher laws (Spritzer, 2003). In the hospital setting, the hospital kosher meals service will undertake this responsibility. All food must be served in specially sealed containers with disposable cutlery and given to the patient without breaking the seal or disturbing the cutlery. In Jewish tradition, meat and milk products must not be mixed. Esme is likely to be experiencing a range of emotions, such as feeling shocked and upset that her religious beliefs have not been sufficiently taken into account. This may lead to feelings of not being valued as a person in her own right. This could also have an effect on her hospital experience in terms of her recovery and ongoing engagement with the healthcare team. Shanique had no previous experience of caring for a Jewish patient and is also likely to be feeling upset, as well as confused and unsure, in this situation due to her lack of knowledge in this particular context. Before Shanique left the bedside, she should have explained to Esme that she was going to get some assistance and that she would return shortly. If, as a student, you are unsure about dietary habits, the easiest way to find out is to ask the patient as they are usually more than willing to explain their specific requirements. You must, however, be clear in your explanation to the patient as to why you are asking for the information so as not to seem intrusive. If you do not feel confident enough to ask the patient, think of ways in which you can build up your confidence in this aspect. This could include keeping a diary of personal reflections or critical incidents on your encounters with people from different cultures (Lonneman, 2015). You could communicate with your practice assessor as well as researching relevant resources to improve your current level of knowledge and understanding. During the initial patient assessment, information on Esme's religious, cultural or spiritual beliefs, as well as contact details of her rabbi, should have been collected and documented. In a situation such as this, contact with the rabbi will be helpful. Personal preferences in line with religious values must be respected in order to provide care that preserves and promotes human dignity (Cheraghi et al., 2014). The last couple of years have seen an increase in the number of people who identify as vegans. While this lifestyle choice may not have a religious foundation, it is nonetheless very important to those individuals who subscribe to this diet. A lifestyle choice must be respected in the same way as a religious observance, and, as a nurse, failure to do this would be disrespectful to a patient's values and beliefs. As you can now understand, due to a lack of knowledge, the result of inadequate nutritional intake will have repercussions on health and the delivery of individualised patient care. This calls for sensitivity and belies the need to ensure a holistic cultural patient assessment in which relevant needs are addressed.

Activity 4.6 Decision-making and leadership (p88)

Nada will need to be sensitive when discussing the issue of vaccination administration given that it does contain porcine (a derivative of pork), which is strictly prohibited in Muslim culture. In addition, Bushra, as a Muslim female, may be feeling uncomfortable having had to speak to a male doctor; even though she is not being examined, there may well be feelings of discomfort. Nada will need to allow Bushra the time to speak about her concerns, paying attention to both verbal as well as non-verbal cues. It is important to find out specifically what Bushra wants to know and what she wants to achieve at the end of the discussion. This can help to guide the amount and type of information provided. Nada will need to explain fully to her the ingredients of the nasal flu vaccine and, if appropriate, suggest the possibility of the alternative injection that does not contain any porcine (PHE, 2014a). It may be helpful to contact Bushra's local imam so that he can provide further instruction as to whether or not it is permissible; in some circumstances, it may be. Consideration needs to be made in terms of the benefits of vaccination, which goes against Bushra's religious beliefs. It is also important to take into account any past medical history Jareem might have. Advice should be given to Bushra on aspects of daily living that might be making Jareem more susceptible to colds and flu, such as diet and home environment. Nada could also contact the health visitor and, with permission, access Jareem's records to find out more information. It is important that Bushra's wishes are respected and that she does not feel she is being forced into making decisions with which she is not happy. More information can be provided to Bushra to aid her understanding so that she can make a fully informed decision that does not go against her beliefs. Leaflets should be used, such as *Protecting Your Child against Flu: Information for Parents* (PHE, 2014a), to reinforce what is said during the verbal interaction. At the end of the discussion, Nada should ask Bushra to recall what she has been told to ensure clarity and understanding. However, it is important to ascertain Bushra's level of literacy as this will impact on the processing of information she is given. Nada should have a discussion with Dr Oros to advise him of the outcome of the consultation and also to explain cultural variations, such as Bushra's lack of engagement, if he is unaware of these. As an observer, in your capacity as a student, you need to examine your own cultural beliefs and how they fit in with the cultural differences highlighted in the scenario. You can reflect on the situation and discuss the various issues raised with your practice assessor. The Public Health England guidance on the use of the nasal vaccine also provides helpful information for health service workers (PHE, 2014b).

Further reading

Barrett, D., Wilson, B. and Woollands, A. (2019) *Care Planning: A Guide for Nurses* (3rd edn). London: Routledge.

Chapter 3 gives the reader underpinning theory in relation to the activities of living model.

Christiansen, A., O'Brien, M.R., Kirton, J.A., Zubairu, K. and Bray, L. (2015) Delivering compassionate care: the enablers and barriers. *British Journal of Nursing*, 24(16): 833–7.

The findings of a study conducted to ascertain the understanding of healthcare staff and pre-registered students of the term 'compassion'.

Department of Health (2009) *Religion or Belief: A Practical Guide for the NHS*. Available at: https://webarchive.nationalarchives.gov.uk/20130123195548/http://www.dh.gov.uk/en/ Publicationsandstatistics/Publications/PublicationsPolicyAndGuidance/DH_093133 (accessed 30 January 2019).

An informative guide on the practicalities for healthcare providers to take into account patient and staff religious and spiritual beliefs.

Douglas, M.K., Rosenkoetter, M., Pacquiao, D.F., Callister, L.C., Hattar-Pollara, M., Lauderdale, J., et al. (2014) Guidelines for implementing culturally competent nursing care. *Journal of Transcultural Nursing*, 25(2): 109–21.

This article provides the reader with background information on the concept of culturally competent care.

Holland, K. (2018) *Cultural Awareness in Nursing and Health Care: An Introductory Text* (3rd edn). London: Routledge.

This is an informed and easy-to-read textbook that provides a good foundation for the reader to explore the concept of cultural awareness.

Papadopoulos, I. (2014) *The Papadopoulos Model for Developing Culturally Competent Compassion in Healthcare Professionals*. Available at: www.youtube.com/watch?v=zjKzO94TevA (accessed 3 February 2019).

This is a short YouTube video that provides an overview of the components of the model.

Quinn, B. (2018) Spiritual care is not as complex as we may think. *Nursing Standard*, 33(9): 69–70.

A short feature article that explores the need for nurses and other healthcare workers to be skilled in delivering spiritual care.

Rogers, M. and Wattis, J. (2015) Spirituality in nursing practice. *Nursing Standard*, 29(39): 51–7.

An informative article that explores the relevance of spirituality in nursing in order to equip staff to deliver care that encompasses a recognition of the essential nature of spirituality to some of the patients with whom we may come into contact.

Sartori, P. (2010) Spirituality 2: exploring how to address patients' spiritual needs in practice. *Nursing Times*, 106(29): 23–5.

An informed article on the need for nurses to be confident in the delivery of spiritual care to patients.

The Evidence Centre (2013) *Content Analysis of 'Patient Opinion' Website Stories about Nurse Attitudes and Behaviours*. Available at: www.careopinion.org.uk/resources/blog-resources/1-files/rcn-professional-attitudes-behaviours-patient-opinion-stories-report.pdf (accessed 11 August 2018).

This organisation, along with the RCN, conducted a study to explore the experiences of patients and relatives in relation to the attitudes and behaviours of nurses with whom they came into contact.

Useful websites

Cultural Competence: e-Learning for Healthcare

www.e-lfh.org.uk/programmes/cultural-competence

This is a new e-learning tool published by Health Education England to assist healthcare professionals in developing their knowledge and skill in aspects around culture and health. You will have to register on the site, unless you already have an account with e-Learning for Healthcare.

Chapter 5

Assessing the needs of diverse patients

Mariama Seray-Wurie and Beverley Brathwaite

NMC Standards of Proficiency for Registered Nurses

This chapter will address the following platforms and proficiencies:

Platform 1: Being an accountable professional

1.4 demonstrate an understanding of, and the ability to challenge, discriminatory behaviour.

1.9 understand the need to base all decisions regarding care and interventions on people's needs and preferences, recognising and addressing any personal and external factors that may unduly influence your decisions.

1.14 provide and promote non-discriminatory, person-centred and sensitive care at all times, reflecting on people's values and beliefs, diverse backgrounds, cultural characteristics, language requirements, needs and preferences, taking account of any need for adjustments.

Platform 2: Promoting health and preventing ill health

2.2 demonstrate knowledge of epidemiology, demography, genomics and the wider determinants of health, illness and wellbeing and apply this to an understanding of global patterns of health and wellbeing outcomes.

2.3 understand the factors that may lead to inequalities in health outcomes.

2.10 provide information in accessible ways to help people understand and make decisions about their health, life choices, illness and care.

Platform 3: Assessing needs and planning care

3.4 understand and apply a person-centred approach to nursing care, demonstrating shared assessment, planning, decision making and goal setting when working with people, their families, communities and populations of all ages.

3.5 demonstrate the ability to accurately process all information gathered during the assessment process to identify needs for individualised nursing care and develop person-centred evidence-based plans for nursing interventions with agreed goals.

Platform 4: Providing and evaluating care

4.1 demonstrate and apply an understanding of what is important to people and how to use this knowledge to ensure their needs for safety, dignity, privacy, comfort and sleep can be met, acting as a role model for others in providing evidence based person-centred care.

4.2 work in partnership with people to encourage shared decision making in order to support individuals, their families and carers to manage their own care when appropriate.

Platform 7: Coordinating care

7.1 understand and apply the principles of partnership, collaboration and inter-agency working across all relevant sectors.

Chapter aims

After reading this chapter, you will be able to:

*   examine the impact of diverse cultural influences affecting health beliefs and perceptions of illness on those in your care;
*   reflect on your own beliefs about health and illness, diversity and culture, and how this may influence your assessment and perception of an individual in your care; and
*   describe key techniques that can be utilised when assessing an individual in your care to ensure recognition of diversity and avoidance of assumptions.

Introduction

Scenario

You and some fellow student nurses are going to a workshop on diversity in the NHS organised by the hospital where you are attending practice placement. The manager on the ward suggests that you go 'as you might find it useful'. The head of nursing starts off the workshop with the following quote, and asks everyone in attendance if they think this happens in their clinical areas, as well as if anyone can give an example of this:

The NHS provides a comprehensive service, available to all irrespective of gender, race, disability, age, sexual orientation, religion, belief, gender reassignment, pregnancy

(Continued)

(Continued)

and maternity or marital or civil partnership status. The service is designed to improve, prevent, diagnose and treat both physical and mental health problems with equal regard. It has a duty to each and every individual that it serves and must respect their human rights. At the same time, it has a wider social duty to promote equality through the services it provides and to pay particular attention to groups or sections of society where improvements in health and life expectancy are not keeping pace with the rest of the population.

(Department of Health, 2015a)

There is silence in the room of over 50 people from varying departments in the hospital.

It can be difficult to place yourself within the larger context of the NHS, and this could be the reason for the silence. The above scenario and quote used is the first principle stated in the NHS Constitution outlining the need to provide a service to all, and within this statement there is an acknowledgement of diversity.

Part of the acknowledgement of diversity within healthcare is about appreciating how an individual perceives health and illness and influencing factors on these phenomena. Nursing has a pivotal role in the delivery of care within the NHS and users of the service will at some point need to have an assessment undertaken by a nurse. Your own views of diversity, health and illness, and your culture will influence to some extent how you deliver care as nurses are from diverse backgrounds. Assessment and care planning is one of the principles in the NMC standards (NMC, 2018), and in line with the code it is a requirement to treat people as individuals, avoid making assumptions, recognising diversity and individual choice (NMC, 2015).

This chapter will allow you to explore your own perceptions of health and illness, diversity, and culture, as your personal understanding of these issues is pivotal in the assessment and planning of care to ensure that your own beliefs do not influence care in an inappropriate way. A significant part of the nurse's role involves working with diverse groups, individuals and families in a variety of healthcare settings. There are many challenges when working with a diverse patient group with different cultures as the individual will have their own health belief systems that may be influenced by their culture, religion, age, gender or sexuality.

This chapter will also examine how personal beliefs from the patient perspective influence health and illness, and how these may not always correspond with Western medicine and the biomedical approach to care. It will address concepts around cultural competency, and the final part of the chapter will focus on exploring ways to ensure equality and inclusivity when assessing and planning care with diverse patient groups.

Why can assessment be complex when managing diverse and culturally different patients?

Assessment in the context of healthcare is a complex process that is completed by a registered nurse, and, as a student, you will be supervised carrying out this activity. It is not just a one-off process as it will be an activity that continues throughout the relationship between you, as a nurse, with the patient/service user and their family where applicable. It is the first step that is undertaken in order to plan care, and as such the assessment needs to be able to capture a detailed representation of the individual that highlights their needs in the time of illness, but also give insight into their beliefs and perception of their health and illness. To undertake this activity, as a nurse, you have to be able to utilise good communication skills such as good questioning technique and listening skills, be observant to responses and body language, and have an open mind and not be judgemental. It is vital that all aspects of the individual's health and illness are explored to formulate a plan of care that will address the needs of the individual and their family where applicable. The process can be described as doing detective work, and as such, even though you may rely on scientific knowledge of the health problem and your own instinctive beliefs, using these solely would result in key problems not being identified correctly or being missed. An assessment in all cases needs to be holistic, addressing physical, psychological and sociological aspects of care and how health has been affected as a result of the illness. This will also ensure that, as a nurse, you explore the individual's perception of how they feel about their health/illness and influencing factors. Individuals and families will conceptualise illness and how it is treated in different ways; this may not be congruent with your expectations, which may possibly lead to you, as a nurse, being prejudiced or judgemental by not recognising or understanding these differing influences. It is therefore relevant for you, as a student, to reflect on some of your own beliefs, values and culture to explore how this could possibly influence negatively or even positively how you assess individuals from diverse backgrounds. To do this, you will need to address reflective learning as in Activity 5.1.

Activity 5.1   Reflection

In Chapter 2, diversity, culture and concepts of health were addressed. Reflecting on your clinical experiences to date, consider an episode of care that you were involved in with an individual of a different background to yourself (and potentially their family). Consider gender, race, disability, age, sexual orientation, religion, belief and gender reassignment. Was there an element during your interactions that made you reflect on their diversity

(Continued)

(Continued)

and culture as an influencing factor that determined how they responded to their illness?

Did you find it difficult to work with them, and did this encounter influence your ideas about diversity and culture?

On completion of your reflection, visit the following link (Flowers, 2014) and use the cultural awareness assessment tool in Table 3:

http://citeseerx.ist.psu.edu/viewdoc/download?doi=10.1.1.571.300&re p=rep1&type=pdf

As this answer is based on your own observation, there is no outline answer at the end of the chapter.

Now that you have thought about your cultural awareness, let us look at how it impacts nursing assessment and care delivery. This will be followed by some scenarios to get you to link in 'real-life' situations.

Cultural awareness

Just learning about other cultures does not always equate to having cultural awareness as a nurse. To develop cultural awareness, self-examination and understanding of one's own cultural beliefs and values related to healthcare and the profession is key. The cultural awareness assessment tool (Flowers, 2014), if answered honestly, will provide this insight to explore your own prejudices and biased views of others based on the score obtained.

An individual may respond to illness the way they do because of their cultural background or in response to how they may have been treated in the past because of their cultural diversity. This may have occurred from a nurse or any other healthcare professional due to a lack of awareness of cultural practices other than their own, or a lack of appreciation of the diversity of individuals and making assumptions. It is an expectation that nurses are able to assess and plan care that is clinically safe and culturally sensitive. However, when undertaking an activity such as assessment, the outcome may be an incorrect interpretation of the individual's needs or becoming frustrated with the individual or their family if there is lack of cultural sensitivity or appreciation of diversity. This goes against Platform 1, 'Being an accountable professional', which states that registered nurses act in the best interests of people, putting them first and providing nursing care that is person-centred, safe and compassionate (NMC, 2018).

The beliefs of the individual play a significant role when assessing and planning care to foster partnership with the individual and their family where relevant. The consensus within nursing about those who enter the profession is the desire to help people (RCN, 2010). From Activity 5.1, you should have recognised that even though, as a student nurse, you are compassionate and care for your patients with good intentions, your personal background, culture, education, race, gender, sexual orientation, age or religion have influenced, and always will influence, to some extent, how you deliver nursing care. You may at this stage, at the start of your career as a student, find these thoughts challenging as you may feel that you are not providing the best care due to your own beliefs. These are occurrences that are experienced with registered nurses such as your practice supervisor too, and the RCN (2010) acknowledges these behaviours in nurses. However, it is not always a negative attribute if you are aware of how your beliefs influence the nursing care you give and the potential of how it may affect the way you see the patient as an individual. Their health condition, both mental as well as physical, and the care they require should not be impacted on negatively, and appropriate action should be taken to avoid this.

Scenario 1

A health visitor is working with the Bada family, who have settled in the UK as refugees. Their eldest child, Yasmin, has severe physical and developmental delays as a result of lack of oxygen at birth. The health visitor would like, with the consent of the parents, to refer the child for an intensive physiotherapy and occupational health programme that would help her to become more independent. The parents, Joseph and Lucy, are declining to give consent as they state it is their duty to care for Yasmin as they believe that the condition of the child is punishment for conceiving her before they were married, and as such it is their burden to care for her. The nurse is very upset with the parents as she feels they are not acting in the best interest of the child.

Scenario 2

Ms Tran arrives in the urgent care centre with her 12-year-old son, Giang. She is Vietnamese and does not speak English, but her child does, and he is interpreting for his mother. Ms Tran has severe abdominal pain and vaginal bleeding. She is clutching her lower abdomen and appears visibly distressed, as does the child, who states he is scared that something will happen to his mother. The nurse who is assigned to the case informs Giang that she is going to get an interpreter so that she can assess the mother, and in the meantime she will have him go to the play area and wait. The mother and child both become very upset as the mother does not want the child to leave her.

Scenario 3

Lizzy, age 42, is an inpatient on the medical ward. She has expressed concern about her partner's ability to care for her children and how she will manage at home when she is discharged. The nurse managing her care suggests that a discharge meeting is organised involving the family and offers to contact her husband. The nurse also states that perhaps Lizzy's mother, Lesley, who has called daily to enquire how she is, be involved in the meeting. Lizzy at that point informs the nurse that Lesley is her partner.

Scenario 4

Errol, age 58, has a long history of mental health problems and Type 2 diabetes. He is known to the community mental health services as he is on medication that is supervised by them. He is divorced and lives alone in a council flat. He has lost sensation in his lower limbs and has sustained a burn injury to the sole of his left foot from a hot water bottle. He has not had the wound assessed by a health professional as he dressed it himself. The community mental health services, on their visit, decide to quickly assess the wound, and on taking off the bandage discover a picture of St Francis of Assisi covered in plastic between the layers of the bandage. Errol describes the picture as a relic that can prevent or positively influence life's problems, and that St Francis is known for healing animals and people; therefore, having the picture in the dressing will help the wound to heal.

Scenario 5

Krishnan, age 37, has recently been diagnosed with chronic renal failure. He has started peritoneal dialysis, and as part of his management, maintaining adequate protein intake is an essential part of his ongoing treatment, of which animal protein is the recommended source. Krishnan is Hindu by religion and has eaten chicken and eggs all his life. However, since the diagnosis, he has decided to become vegetarian as he wants to become a good Hindu so that God will help him with his ordeal. He states that not eating meat is a more devout way of life and one he wishes to follow.

Looking at these scenarios, you should now start to have an awareness of the complexities involved when undertaking patient assessment with diverse patient groups

Activity 5.2 Critical thinking

How would you respond to the scenarios described above and why?

This is an activity to be done from your perspective, based on your personal values and beliefs; therefore, there is no outline answer at the end of the chapter. However, there are some valuable ideas to consider, outlined at the end of the chapter.

and their beliefs. From Activity 5.1, you should be able to conclude that the individuals and their families have their unique identity, influenced by how they see themselves with regard to personal background, culture, education, race, gender, sexual orientation, age or religion. Therefore, as a nurse, focusing on only one aspect of their identity is counterproductive when undertaking assessment and planning of care as there is the potential for you to stereotype. Although stereotypes can be positive as well as negative, from the negative perspective, if you have a stereotypical view of the individual in your care, it can hinder communication (Jandt and Jandt, 2018) and create bias, which in turn will cause barriers in the partnership working relationship with your patient. When there are barriers, the outcome will be a plan of care that does not meet the needs of the individual, and possibly care that is substandard as a result of the nurse and other health professionals not factoring in the wider cultural and diverse influences (Papadopoulos, 2006). In addition to the NMC standards and the NMC code, which clearly state the need to recognise and respect difference, as a student, you must also be aware of relevant legislation that is key with regard to the commitment to promote equality and stop unlawful racial discrimination. This is the Equality Act 2010, which brought together several pieces of legislation together as one Act, providing a legal framework that is easier to understand to protect the rights of individuals and promote equal opportunity for all. With regard to nursing practice, the Equality Act 2010 is relevant as the services that have to be provided in any healthcare setting, whether primary or acute, must not treat all individuals as the same, but recognise diversity to meet individuals' needs. As a nurse, it is therefore vital to be aware of individual differences (Griffith, 2009). It can be argued that it is not possible for the nurse to understand and be competent in assessment and planning of care for every diverse group as the UK is very ethnically diverse, with a significant LGBTQ population and a growing elderly population, and with improvements in healthcare provision, people with disabilities and long-term conditions are living longer. However, this should not deter you, as identified by O'Hagan (2001), who advocates that 'how you approach' someone who is from a different culture is more important than being highly knowledgeable about the differences.

Having got some clarity of the impact of personal beliefs and the need to appreciate difference, we can now consider the patient and family perspective in Activity 5.3.

Activity 5.3   Critical thinking

Now look again at the five previous scenarios. What factors do you think influence perceptions of illness from the patient and family perspective, and what is the relevance of this when assessing an individual?

Thinking about the patient's perspective can only help with being able to make the right clinical decisions with and for the patient.

An outline of what you might find is given at the end of the chapter.

Relevance of patients' beliefs to the assessment process

When assessing a patient, for this to be truly holistic, their culture must be a fundamental part of the assessment process and planning of care, as does an appreciation of the diversity of the patient. This will ensure that the care for the patient is culturally appropriate. Evidence in the literature (Bjarnason et al., 2009; Meddings and Hiath-Cooper, 2008) shows that in situations when care is not culturally appropriate, this leads to an undesirable course of events, from miscommunication to life-threatening incidents.

Understanding of the health beliefs of the individual is key when assessing the patient, as perception of illness and the cause varies by culture and individual preferences, which will influence how you assess and deliver care as a nurse. For care to be inclusive of culture and diversity, it must combine the beliefs, values and attitude of the patient and their family where relevant with the values that are subscribed to within healthcare provision, which tends to be mainly based on Western values and the biomedical model of care. Issues of conflict may arise when a healthcare professional disregards or fails to appreciate other influences outside of the biomedical model and Western practices.

Let us look again at the five scenarios above. You were asked to think of how the nurses responded, which should have again highlighted how personal beliefs and values would have influenced the reaction. You were also asked to think about the scenarios from the patient perspective; Activity 5.2 outlines some of the cultural factors from a patient perspective. The scenarios touch lightly on some factors that influence beliefs in health and illness within diverse patient groups. Individuals will have different views about the origin, causes and best way to treat illness, and, as a nurse, this must be recognised when undertaking patient assessment and applied to all diverse groups. Even a child or young person has their beliefs about illness, and this must be respected. Culture is a clear factor that influences belief; however, it is also key to recognise that even though you may have individuals from the same background, this does not necessarily mean they believe in the same cultural practices, and therefore you should not assume this. Religion, which will be discussed in Chapter 6, influences beliefs regarding health and illness, and again the same principle applies with regard to making assumptions as religion in itself has diverse practices. Going back to scenarios 1 and 3, it is evident that the beliefs held in the scenarios do not match up with what you perceive as a duty of care, as a nurse, but also a lack of awareness or understanding of an individual's customs. Getting to know your patient and the perceptions of their illness is a generic principle that is applied in all aspects of nursing care, and where there are beliefs that may not be congruent with the evidence that clinical practice is based on, it is about working in partnership with the individual to see how their needs can be best met. This is where your listening and observational skills are important when you are undertaking assessment. In addition to the issues of culture and religion, other factors, such as gender, education, socio-economic background, career and family traditions, will influence an individual's perception of health and illness (Griffith, 2009). From the assessment and when planning the care, it is about having a balance. This means utilising both the patient's influences and the scientific evidence. It may be that you are of the opinion that the biomedical approach to illness is best, and indeed this may be a fact; however, if the patient and their family do not see it this way, then to address this complexity an egalitarian or open approach needs to be evident. In the past and with biomedical models, a paternalistic approach was taken with patients; however, as the population has grown and become more diverse, other factors that influence health and illness have become very evident, and legislation such as the Equality Act 2010 means that within healthcare settings, care has to be delivered that recognises and supports the equality of all people, taking on board their needs by working in partnership with the patient and their family.

How to ensure equality and inclusivity when assessing and planning care for diverse patient groups

Dr Jean Watson, an American nursing theorist who has written extensively on the theory of nursing and theory of caring (Watson, 1988), talks about nursing being defined by caring. Watson's caring theory focuses on the relational processes that healthcare workers engage with patients' families and each other. In her theory of caring it is core that humans are not treated as objects and that humans cannot be separated from self, other, nature and the larger workforce (Watson, 2008). Emphasis is on the interpersonal process between the healthcare giver and care recipient. Dr Jean Watson's theories on nursing and caring capture the issues that have been discussed so far about the attitude of the nurse and the perception of the patient and their family about health and illness. To provide and promote non-discriminatory, person-centred and sensitive care at all times that reflects on the values, beliefs, diverse backgrounds, cultural characteristics and language requirements as outlined by the NMC (2018), a nurse should be culturally aware, culturally knowledgeable and culturally sensitive in their practice.

Recognising the diverse nature of the users of the health service is the first step. Then understanding their needs should follow to develop the relationship value, and this understanding of needs must be taken into consideration for care to be personalised. However, given the wide range of diverse groups of patients, it is not possible to have an understanding about every diverse group and their cultural practices; therefore, it should be the approach to diversity and cultural differences that is key. When undertaking patient assessment, the outcome is to understand what the patient's needs are. These needs are unique to the patient and will include clinical symptoms that need medical/nursing attention and issues specific to the individual that can affect their care.

When undertaking patient assessment, it is important for you to be prepared to address not just the clinical symptoms, but also the spectrum of demographics and personal characteristics that will influence individual beliefs and responses to health and illness. In Activity 5.2, you should have identified cultural data in the scenarios that are part of the spectrum of demographics and personal characteristics. Williamson and Harrison (2010) identify two approaches defining culture and providing appropriate care, which can be considered as patient assessment in delivering care. Considering that it is an expectation to provide culturally appropriate care, one approach identified is a cognitive approach that focuses on cognitive aspects of culture, traditions, values and beliefs with the assumption that they are shared by those from the same background or group. If this approach is used, it means that you would have to learn about specific cultural groups in relation to these cognitive aspects of culture to be able to assess and provide appropriate care. In addition, with this approach, awareness of your own culture and being able to understand and accept difference is required. Learning as much as you can about how others see health and illness from their perspective may make you more sensitive to individual needs of people from certain groups. However, the downside to this is acceptance that culture is something that is static and that all peoples who subscribe to that culture are the same, which can lead to stereotyping. From your understanding of culture in the earlier chapters, there are differences within cultures, and people do change as they are influenced by other factors that change or adapt their traditions, values and beliefs. The second approach suggested by Williamson and Harrison (2010) is a broader approach. Rather than focusing on cognitive aspects of culture as in learning about customs and beliefs of particular groups to plan appropriate care, the focus is on the individual's social position and how this impacts their health and well-being. This is a more critical approach. The reason why a more critical approach may be appropriate is that it provides insights into the social position and power relationships between the individual and how these influences impact on health. It includes, and is not restricted to, age, gender, sexual orientation, ethnicity or migrant experience, religious/spiritual beliefs, socio-economic status, and disability.

Research summary: assessing patients with dark-pigmented skin

Skin colour matters in health care. Clinicians make decisions based on colour assessments multiple times each day as they gauge tissue perfusion and assess for jaundice, pallor, cyanosis, and the blanch response.

(Everett et al., 2012, p496)

This statement identifies the slow growing field of research on the important practicalities of understanding that not all skin pigmentation is the same, and what is being done to address this. The focus should be on the physiology of the skin, and not the socially constructed attributes connected to skin colour, such as race, ethnicity, culture, religion and language, although research on pressure ulcer assessment finds that making this distinction can be difficult in healthcare, as in society. Oozageer Gunowa et al. (2018) found that detecting pressure damage in people with darker skin tones is mainly focused on ethnicity and race rather than variations in skin pigmentation. This is an unreliable tool to assess skin damage – the patient's skin tone should be the focus of the assessment allowing for individualised care (Oozageer Gunowa et al., 2018). What happens when we do not assess patients with dark-pigmented skin adequately for pressure damage is that erythema and Category 1 pressure ulcers are at higher risk of pressure ulcer development, and they are more likely to go undetected and deteriorate (Baker, 2016; Sullivan, 2014).

Rather than exercising 'color blindness' when assessing and treating patients, practitioners should exercise 'color awareness' by adjusting interventions and assessment techniques using the patients' physiological characteristics rather than depending on racial or ethnic categorization to guide care (Sommers, 2011).

(Everett et al., 2012, p507)

This is an essential point that you need to carry with you when assessing all patients, but particularly those with darker skin tones, when carrying out a visual assessment, whether it be cyanosis or eczema in children (Myers, 2015). It is vital to develop your knowledge on how to assess in other ways, taking into consideration skin pigmentation. In the further reading section, we direct you to resources that will be useful to you in learning what can be done and practising this in your clinical placements.

Cultural competency

Platform 3, 'Assessing needs and planning care' (NMC, 2018), states that the registered nurse should work in partnership with people to develop person-centred care plans that take into account their circumstances, characteristics and preferences. The process for this would start with patient assessment, and during this process you will need to develop the ability to collect relevant data about the presenting problem, which would include objective and subjective data. As part of the data collection to ensure that assessment and planning of care is clinically safe and culturally sensitive, relevant cultural data regarding the problem will be required, and you will need to develop the ability to extract this information from the individual and their family where applicable. For you to do this, you need to be culturally competent, bearing in mind that culture is not only about beliefs and values on race and ethnicity, but other determinants, such as age, gender, education, religion, socio-economic status and occupation, need to be considered.

There are five attributes that define cultural competence that should be demonstrated by nurses during care delivery: cultural awareness, cultural sensitivity, cultural knowledge, cultural skill and dynamic process.

Cultural awareness

Cultural awareness should have emerged from the reflective exercise. In summary, this is about the nurse having self-awareness of their own cultural values, beliefs and practices to better understand the practices of other cultural groups, and where personal stereotypes, biases or assumptions are evident towards other cultures that are seen as different, recognising that these must be explored. Thus, within cultural awareness, the nurse becomes mindful of the different values, beliefs, norms and lifestyles of the individual person and their family where applicable, recognising cultural similarities and differences, as well as the influence of culture to health and its value in nursing care provision.

Cultural sensitivity

Cultural sensitivity is the awareness not to assume that individuals from the same culture are the same as there is diversity within cultures. Appreciation of this diversity is key to achieving mutual learning and develop trust, as well as respecting cultural differences to allow genuine and satisfactory care.

Cultural knowledge

Cultural knowledge is when the nurse has accomplished an educational base to better understand different beliefs, values and behaviours about various cultural groups that they may be presented with in professional practice. Within cultural knowledge, the nurse will know about what are acceptable and unacceptable behaviours when interacting with different cultures in relation to etiquette, communication and diet, to name a few activities. Having this knowledge and understanding when assessing and planning care better prepares the nurse before the encounter. It also means that a better service provision can be achieved.

Cultural skill

Cultural skill is about the ability of the nurse to undertake a cultural assessment that collects relevant cultural data of the current health problem of the individual in a sensitive manner and to incorporate this data into the planning of care accurately. One of the key skills required is effective communication, which is addressed in Chapter 3.

Dynamic process

Dynamic process is about 'becoming culturally competent' as a nurse rather than 'being culturally competent'. As identified earlier within this chapter, it is not possible for the nurse to know about all cultures and the diversity within those cultures. Globalisation and migration mean that nurses will continue to encounter individuals with different cultures from diverse backgrounds. Within these consistent encounters, cultural competence will gradually develop as the striving to provide care continues. Also, cultures change, and people change, and as such cultural competence cannot be a static process where there is no room for ongoing development.

Reflecting back to the previous scenarios, you should be able to see how a nurse can show cultural competence when assessing and managing events in the scenarios. The five attributes are areas that you should develop as you progress and transition throughout your nursing career. Having completed the Activity 5.1, you can see that you may have some of these attributes already and can continue to develop those, or have identified that you do not have any as yet, but you now have a starting point to develop.

Challenges in planning care for diverse patients

Having looked at the attributes when assessing and planning care in the context of culture and diversity, exploration of some of the difficulties you may encounter, as well as the causes, is also key. Look back to Activity 5.1, where you were asked to reflect on a clinical practice experience. The main areas of concern are stereotyping and labelling, as well as acculturation (Flowers, 2014).

Stereotyping is usually done unintentionally, and it involves making generalisations about some aspect of an individual or a group of people. However, not everyone in a specific cultural group has the same attitudes and assumptions to health and illness. As we have seen, there are various factors that can influence attitudes and assumptions when the focus is not on the cognitive aspects of culture. Within different groups, subcultures and variations exist, and just because a person may have the appearance that belongs to a certain culture does not necessarily mean they subscribe to what would be assumed as the 'norms' for that culture. Labels may be based on their ethnicity, age, gender orientation or disease.

Acculturation is another area that can pose challenges. There is an assumption that when an individual or their family has chosen to come to this country, they will integrate and adopt the British culture, modifying their own culture as a result of integration, and in some cases completely adopting British culture. This is not always the case, and there are many incidences where integration has not occurred and individuals have retained their cultural practices. In such incidences, it is important for the nurse to establish how much integration the individual and family have made to belong to British culture. Acculturation will be looked at again in Chapter 7 in relation to religious beliefs.

Key points to remember when assessing

Beliefs about health and illness will vary considerably between different cultures that you encounter and also within any given culture. Do not make assumptions, as looking the same does not mean being the same. There are a range of factors, including ethnicity and place of origin, education, religion, values, gender, age, family, and social status, that will influence the cultural perspective of the individual. As a nurse, when you undertake a patient's assessment and care planning, recognise that your beliefs and values about health for the individual and their family can be quite different from that of your patients. Even though it is possible that the same broad culture is shared, it is still important to value the individual.

To ensure that your assessment and the care you plan are culturally sensitive and meet the needs of the individual who has a different cultural background to yours, you will need to have an understanding of their perspective, which can be gained by asking more questions. The stereotype may not always fit; just because the individual looks different does not infer that they want different. Being culturally aware is one of the key steps you can take to start becoming 'culturally competent'. You can do this by recognising your own preconceptions that you may have when undertaking an assessment activity and aiming not to make assumptions, but instead seeking clarity and checking understanding from the individual and their family where relevant. The process is a lifelong learning activity as it is not possible to be knowledgeable about and understand all cultures and diverse groups. What you can have is an open attitude that *appreciates* the views of others, *behaviour* that validates and respects the cultural beliefs of others, and clear and open *communication* – the A, B and C outlined by Heaslip (2015).

Chapter summary

This chapter has given an overview of the impact of diverse cultural influences affecting one's health beliefs and the perception that illness has through reflection of your own beliefs about culture, diversity, health and illness, allowing for the importance of assessing in the process of care delivery for patients from diverse backgrounds and communities.

Activities: brief outline answers

Activity 5.2   Critical thinking (p101)

Scenario 1

This is about providing culturally sensitive care as everyone has a culture, and to assess and provide appropriate care the nurse must understand their culture, that of the profession, and be sensitive to the biases each individual or the family may bring to the therapeutic relationship.

In this case scenario, the health visitor did not fully understand the initial refusal of treatment by the family, and this would be an issue that they would have reflected on and discussed with colleagues as the family are not conforming to the 'norms' of care. When you then become culturally aware, the health visitor realises that their own personal beliefs and professional values of independence are the cause of upset with the parents' refusal to accept referral to therapies. The health visitor decides to go back and explore with the family their goals for their child. By doing this, they learn that the parents want the child to become stronger and have fewer infections. When the same therapies are described as a means of meeting these goals, the parents are quite willing to participate. The programme was developed to meet goals that the family identified as important.

In-depth knowledge of all cultures is unrealistic, but it is possible to gain a broad understanding of how culture affects beliefs and behaviours. Acquiring cultural knowledge begins with recognition that behaviours and responses viewed one way in one cultural context by the professional may have a different meaning in another cultural context for the individual.

Scenario 2

When carrying out patient assessment where the language barrier is an issue, an interpreter can be essential, as the nurse is responsible for assessing and understanding of the information provided. It is important, as a nurse, to recognise the need for an interpreter, as illustrated in the scenario. Reliance on the child or other relative to interpret can be convenient for the parent; however, the nurse has to be sensitive to the needs of the mother and child. Given the nature of the presenting symptoms, both mother and son may feel uncomfortable talking about the current health issues, which may compromise the accuracy when taking the history. An interpreter, preferably female, should be quite urgently sought for the assessment to be thorough and accurate. The nurse will also need to address the child's concerns and fears in an appropriate manner. It would be an exceptional case if the child is used to interpret, and in cases where a family member is used to interpret, as a nurse, you must carefully evaluate each situation on an ongoing basis as you do not want the assessment to be inaccurate.

Scenario 3

This is about working in partnership with the patient to develop a comprehensive plan of care that is individual and inclusive of the influence of the patient's culture and other influencing factors, such as family dynamics and roles within the family. In this scenario, the nurse has made an assumption about family dynamics, assuming that the partner is male and the mother is supportive to the entire family. The issue of family, even with current laws and openness, can be sensitive for many couples who are LGBTQ. For some, 'family' is often their chosen 'family' as opposed to their bloodline. Use of the word 'partner' and asking the patient who they wish to choose for a family meeting will show openness and a non-judgemental attitude from the nurse.

Scenario 4

The focus of this scenario is about establishing mutual goals and being creative with a commitment to client-focused care, which are key attributes relevant for integrating cultural preferences into the plan of care. This is known as culture care preservation (Leininger, 1988). Having assessed the wound and taking into consideration Errol's preference, the nurse will have to consider the risk of harm depending on the nature of damage the wound has caused, as the nurse will have to decide if further input is required to manage the wound. Although the request is unusual, it does not pose any threat if appropriately cleansed and wrapped in gauze, as it will not be going directly on the wound surface, and the spiritual benefit of the relic to Errol should be recognised.

It is important for physical, emotional and spiritual health to be able to integrate preference of the individual in the assessment and plan of care when there is no risk of harm to the individual or others. This does not mean that, as a nurse, you agree with or endorse the practice for the individual or for others.

Scenario 5

This scenario is about the culture care re-patterning approach, whereby the nurse works with the patient to develop new approaches beyond the patient's normal way of doing things. In this case, the nurse needs to recognise that during times of crisis, such as ill health, a patient may revert to more traditional beliefs. This may differ from a choice taken prior to becoming ill and not following through fully. In this case, the sudden change in dietary practice has to be established. Having established this, the focus or goal is not to change Krishnan's beliefs, but to increase his choices and how to achieve adequate protein intake. It would be necessary, following assessment, to involve the dietician to teach him ways of how he can increase his protein intake from vegetarian sources. His spiritual needs should also be addressed by involving a Hindu priest; this is an effective way of addressing and providing him with insight into resuming animal protein if he so chooses. Ultimately, though, the choice will be his.

Activity 5.3   Critical thinking (p102)

1. Role of family (roles of members, hierarchy, key decision-maker)
2. Role of the wider community with which they associate
3. Religion (impact on diet, beliefs about illness, treatment)
4. Personal views on health and wellness
5. Personal views on death and dying
6. Eastern/Western/alternative/traditional medicine
7. Beliefs about causes and treatments of illness, disease (physical and mental)
8. Gender roles and relationships and position within society
9. Sexuality, fertility and childbirth
10. Food beliefs and diet
11. Socio-economic factors or status
12. Level of education

Further reading

Baker, M. (2016) Detecting pressure damage in people with darkly pigmented skin. *Wound Essentials*, 11(1): 28–31.

A good practical guide at how to assess a patient with darker skin tone.

Catalano, J.T. (2015) *Nursing Now! Today's Issues, Tomorrow's Trends.* Philadelphia, PA: FA Davis.

Chapter 22 in this book has an American perspective, but does give good insight into issues that impact on nursing globally.

Oozageer Gunowa, N., Hutchinson, M., Brooke, J. and Jackson, D. (2018) Pressure injuries in people with darker skin tones: a literature review. *Journal of Clinical Nursing,* 27(17–18): 3266–75.

A comprehensive review of the evidence that is currently out there on this topic. A must-read.

Papadopoulos, I. (2018) *Culturally Competent Compassion: A Guide for Healthcare Students and Practitioners.* London: Routledge.

This book gives a well-structured, up-to-date guide on culturally competent care that is well worth reading. Chapter 4, on health and illness in multicultural societies, is particularly useful.

Useful websites

Intercultural Education of Nurses and Health Professionals in Europe (IENE)

http://ieneproject.eu/mooc.php

This multilingual website addresses nurses and healthcare professionals working in contact with patients with different cultures and languages, and aims to improve the quality of vocational education and training of nurses in Europe.

Chapter 6

Spirituality, death, grief and loss

Beverley Brathwaite

NMC Standards of Proficiency for Registered Nurses

This chapter will address the following platforms and proficiencies:

Platform 2: Promoting health and preventing ill health

2.10 provide information in accessible ways to help people understand and make decisions about their health, life choices, illness and care.

Platform 3: Assessing needs and planning care

3.4 understand and apply a person-centred approach to nursing care, demonstrating shared assessment, planning, decision making and goal setting when working with people, their families, communities and populations of all ages.

3.14 identify and assess the needs of people and families for care at the end of life, including requirements for palliative care and decision making related to their treatment and care preferences.

3.16 demonstrate knowledge of when and how to refer people safely to other professionals or services for clinical intervention or support.

Platform 4: Providing and evaluating care

4.4 demonstrate the knowledge and skills required to support people with commonly encountered mental health, behavioural, cognitive and learning challenges, and act as a role model for others in providing high quality nursing interventions to meet people's needs.

Chapter aims

After reading this chapter, you will be able to:

- demonstrate what death means to different communities in the UK and how to support patients;

- demonstrate an awareness of the differences and commonalities between spirituality and religion;
- understand the needs of end-of-life care for diverse patients;
- identify the experiences of death, grief and loss from differing religious and cultural perspectives; and
- look at how, as healthcare professionals, we use religion and spirituality appropriately in care delivery.

Introduction

Case study: Imposing religious beliefs

A nurse at a Kent hospital was dismissed and then placed under restrictions for imposing her religious beliefs on patients, and in particular giving her personal Bible to a patient. The nurse argued that she hadn't intended to impose her beliefs, and after a hearing at the NMC in 2018 the restrictions were lifted, and she is now able to practise unrestricted. She said, 'I didn't expect to be sacked so I was shocked. This means so much to me because I can go back to the profession I love'.

(adapted from BBC News, 2018)

This unfortunate situation highlights how the best religious intentions can lead to significant penalties for a registered nurse. There are many positions that can be taken regarding what took place and the initial and final outcome for the registered nurse in the case study; here, the focus is on religion and the nurse–patient relationship. There was no malice intended from the nurse; she only wished to use her religion to help her patients. However, we are not all the same, and patients differ in how much they wish religion and spiritualty to be incorporated into the care they receive. The RCN (2011) says 'the nursing profession needs to explore and debate the boundaries that exist between personal belief and professional practice' (p5) and needs to be clear about how they express their beliefs in their own lives, whether through doctrine, ritual or membership of a religious community. Such clarity is essential if they are to remain objective when assessing, planning and delivering holistic patient care. This is supported by Clarridge (2017), who discusses that nurses need to be aware of their own beliefs and values in order to best meet the spiritual care needs of patients, as well as the need for objectivity while providing support to the patient and not allowing their own values and beliefs to impinge upon or influence the patient in any way.

Moving away from personal interactions to healthcare more broadly, the following quotation addresses the varied perspectives that are out there about religion and healthcare:

There are many people who think religion is integral to health care. There are many others who think religion has no place in a health care setting. For some people religion is a part of who they are and informs their decisions and actions. For others it is something they want no part of – these people find it intrusive or even offensive to have spirituality or denominational religion introduced into health care. We wondered how do religion and health care mix? Should they mix? How does a doctor or nurse know when to introduce religion into their practice?

(*Narrative Inquiry in Bioethics* Editors, 2014, p189)

This chapter will look at these issues surrounding religion, healthcare professionals and care delivery. We will discuss how the nurse practitioner must take into consideration the differing religious faiths and spiritual needs of our diverse patients. The chapter will then discuss the complex concepts of religion, spirituality and faith, and how they are combined into healthcare and nursing. Finally, we will examine how various communities view religion, death, grief and end-of-life care, and how we, as healthcare professionals, can use their and our understanding of these issues to deliver high-quality care at one of the most sensitive times in a person's life journey.

Religion, spirituality and faith discussions in nursing and healthcare

According to the 2011 census for England and Wales, the five largest religions are Christianity (33.2 million followers, 59.3 per cent), Islam (2.7 million followers, 4.4 per cent), Hinduism (817,000 followers, 1.5 per cent), Sikhism (420,000 followers, 0.8 per cent) and Judaism (263,000 followers, 0.5 per cent). In 2011, London was the most diverse region, with the highest proportion of people identifying themselves as Muslim, Buddhist, Hindu and Jewish. The North East and North West had the highest proportion of Christians, and Wales had the highest proportion of people reporting no religion (ONS, 2012). 'Religion', 'spirituality', 'faith' and 'belief' are terms used separately or in varied combinations in the literature and clinical practice. It is safe to say that trying to define them is particularly difficult, and what will be done here is an observation of the evidence base 'debate' around the meaning of these terms. McSherry and Jamieson (2011) claim that, as nurses, we should question these terms to encourage a greater understanding of what they mean for the patient and for nursing as a profession when delivering care. Pesut (2016) argues that religious practices *inform* spiritual practices, and what makes them different is that they are practised separately from organised religion. This agrees with McSherry and Jamieson's (2011) argument that the relationship between religious theory and spiritual theory should not be dealt with in a simplistic way by nursing practitioners. Timmins and Caldeira (2017a) consider the actual day-to-day experience, expression and social effect of these terms, which is more important than any actual definition, as does Reimer-Kirkham (2014), who is more concerned with how we live with religion and spirituality.

Part 2 of the Equality Act 2006 defines 'religion' as 'any religion' and 'belief' as 'any religion or religious or philosophical belief', as opposed to 'any religion, religious belief or similar philosophical belief' (Burford et al., 2009, p8). Here, legislation highlights the difficult task of defining religion and amplifies the strong connection between religion and belief. Therefore, for many people who are religious, spirituality refers to the soul and its protection and nurturing during life. The soul may be considered 'protected' through truthful moral thought and by living as directed through sacred texts such the Bible or Koran. This is referred to as having faith (Oman, 2011).

Chopra (2012) considers spirituality being about the individual's belief system, world view, and the relationship they have with a transcendent authority, as defined by the faith or by the individual respecting sacred texts, if appropriate, or as expressed by the individual themselves giving meaning to all the important aspects of their life. One example would be purpose, which guides them through every aspect of their lives and helps them to navigate between what is known/science and unknown/beyond science. It may appear that the known/science is on one side and the unknown/beyond science is on another, and that the two cannot be bought together. For Chopra (2012), however, spirituality complements science, enabling people to be sure of themselves and have confidence in the life choices that they make.

Murray and Zentner (1989) suggest that spirituality is a universal phenomenon that is a deeply personal, sensitive, frequently hidden area of human existence that relates to all people, those with a religious belief and those with none. In a general sense, religion carries transcendent (sacred) and social dimensions, with its practice typically occurring through relatively formal social institutions such as a church, temple, mosque or gurdwara. Spirituality is more about how a person expresses their values or beliefs; as Timmins and Caldeira (2017b) suggest, someone might self-identify as 'religious', 'spiritual', 'both' or 'neither':

> *Religion and spirituality may largely service the same psychological function and the different terms that people use themselves may be a matter of personal preference or style. Therefore, people call themselves religious and spiritual, religious but not spiritual, spiritual but not religious, neither spiritual nor religious, and, very interestingly, a hair-splitting blend of religious spirituality plus nonreligion.*

> (p50)

These terms are regularly used interchangeably. The key point to acknowledge here is that many of your patients will believe in something, and this may be based on an organised religion or not, but an acknowledgement of this as part of your assessment is necessary.

Diverse communities, religion and spirituality

How, then, do we, as nurses, think about incorporating religion and spirituality in our patient care, with diverse religious beliefs and cultural preferences around care delivery?

NHS Scotland Chaplaincy Services (2007) have seven standards that strategically outline how religious and spiritual needs can be addressed across healthcare systems, from access to services, education and training, to staff support.

Activity 6.1 requires you to do two things: (1) look at the spirituality and religion discussion, specifically in relation to clinical practice and care; and (2) consider the importance of incorporating differing religious and cultural points of view and beliefs when caring for patients from diverse backgrounds.

Activity 6.1   Critical thinking

Go to NHS Education for Scotland by following the below link.

www.nes.scot.nhs.uk/education-and-training/by-discipline/spiritual-care/about-spiritual-care/publications/standards-for-nhsscotland-chaplaincy-services.aspx

Read Standards 1 and 3. What changes might your make to your practice based on this information?

An outline of what you might find is given at the end of chapter.

The importance of religious and spiritual care for our patients, as well as what can be done to assure that these needs for our patients are met, is outlined in the NHS Education for Scotland standards on chaplaincy services (NHS Scotland Chaplaincy Services, 2007). This is practical and helpful guidance on how you can incorporate good practice around religion and spirituality. We will now look at the discussion around healthcare, nursing, religion and spirituality, with a focus on professional bodies.

The NMC code of conduct states the following:

> *Carry out comprehensive, systematic nursing assessments that take account of relevant physical, social, cultural, psychological, spiritual, genetic and environmental factors, in partnership with service users and others through interaction, observation and measurement.*

> (NMC, 2015, p8)

Evidently, spirituality is important to nursing and patient care as it has been clearly articulated in the code of conduct for nursing. This does highlight that currently, spirituality takes precedence over religion in the current nursing establishment. However, religion has had a strong connection to nursing and healthcare from its beginning. Religious communities such as nuns cared for the sick, destitute and dying. Then the formation of the National Health Service (NHS) witnessed a decline in these religious connections as health and welfare provision became state-controlled and secular (Ramezani et al., 2014).

Within the nursing literature, Ramezani et al. (2014) discuss ideas of spirituality focusing on enhancing patients' spiritual well-being. The emphasis is on patient-centred care and ensuring that, as nurses, we consider all aspects of the patient experience of health in order to deliver high-quality nursing care.

The RCN surveyed its nursing members to discover what was happening out in practice and how nurses were engaging with spirituality and religion. What follows is a breakdown of key points.

The Royal College of Nursing spirituality survey: categories and aims

Exploration and analysis

Discover and explore RCN members' understanding of, and attitudes towards, the concepts of spirituality and spiritual care.

Prevalence and practice

Identify whether the spiritual needs of patients are recognised by RCN members in the delivery of nursing care.

Education and training

Establish whether RCN members feel that they receive sufficient education and training to enable them to effectively meet patients'/clients' spiritual needs.

Religious belief and spirituality

Explore the associations that may exist between religious belief and RCN members' understandings of spirituality and the provision of spiritual care.

Table 6.1 The Royal College of Nursing spirituality survey
Source: RCN (2011, p6)

As you can see in Table 6.1, the focus of the RCN's enquiry was to find out more about spirituality, but religion was also part of the survey, emphasising the connection between spirituality and religion. Over 4,000 RCN members participated in the survey, and the results did identify some important points. In culturally and ethnically diverse, learning disability and LGBTQ communities, there is evidence that repeatedly shows that these groups do not receive care equitably, and the findings here indicate what a large number of nurses consider to be important in providing care by identifying how spirituality guides them in their practice. Analysing the data, McSherry and Jamieson (2011) identified the following:

1. *Spiritual care is an integral and fundamental aspect of nursing care which may be indistinguishable from psychosocial care.*

2. *Spiritual care concerns the personal caring qualities and attributes of the nurse such as showing care, compassion, cheerfulness and kindness in their communication and interaction with patients.*

3. *Respecting privacy and dignity and supporting individuals with their cultural and religious beliefs are central to the delivery of spiritual care.*

4. *Nurses were aware of the need to refer to and involve the patients' own religious/spiritual leader if necessary.*

5. *Nurses, chaplains, patients, family and friends and other health care professionals were responsible for providing spiritual care.*

6. *Nurses do not feel that they have a monopoly with regard to spiritual care and they are also aware of the need to liaise and collaborate with other health care professionals such as chaplains to support patients in this area.*

(pp1761–2)

These findings indicate the importance that spirituality plays in key aspects of delivering quality nursing care. However, as important as spirituality is, nurses find it challenging to give spiritual care and understand it:

> *Spiritual care is the collection of practices and behaviours that are generally seen as aimed towards helping someone to find spiritual well-being so that they have the strength and resilience to cope with the crisis they are in.*

(Clarke, 2016, p312)

This is so important when looking after patients from diverse backgrounds. These highlighted findings indicate that nursing care can impact more significantly on the aforementioned diverse communities. As previously discussed (see Chapters 1 and 2), evidence suggests that equity of treatment from healthcare professionals in these aspects of care delivery are poorer than with the general population.

However, it must not be underestimated how much religion has a symbiotic relationship with spirituality, and never more so with patients from diverse religious and cultural backgrounds. Religion is central to the lives of many people of African and Caribbean descent in the UK, most likely Christianity (Burrell, 2019). Pesut (2016) suggests that the separation between theories of religion and theories of spirituality does not help the day-to-day lives of nurses in practice. Like many aspects of health, there should be a multidisciplinary approach to meet the specific needs of the patient (McSherry and Jamieson, 2011; RCN, 2010). There needs to be an awareness on the part of nurses of diverse patients' religion, spirituality, faith and health beliefs, rituals, practices, and observances in all healthcare settings. Being alert to patients' beliefs is vital, because these can have a major bearing on their health, both physical and psychological, as well as treatment (Burrell, 2019; Timmins and Caldeira, 2017a).

Religion does not exist in a vacuum; it is socially and historically rooted in society and healthcare, changes over time, and has a powerful shared effect (Pesut, 2016; RCN, 2010).

The same can be said of the history of differing ethnic and cultural communities in the UK. It can be easy to focus solely on Christianity as it remains the most popular religion in England and Wales, with 59.3 per cent of the population identifying themselves as Christian (ONS, 2012). However, this would miss out on religious practices of differing ethnicities and cultural communities, as well as the impact that religion has on healthcare decision-making, reaction to distress, and handling and internalising illness. Without this knowledge and understanding that comes from religion, nurses may find it challenging to provide spiritual care that is sympathetic to patients' values and beliefs (Pesut, 2016).

Think about your own religious, spiritual or cultural background. These are not some separate parts of you, as a healthcare professional. While you may share the same religion as a patient, this does not mean that you know what the patient wants or that they will necessarily share the same beliefs (Mendes, 2015). An acknowledgement and knowledge of your patient's religious, spiritual and cultural beliefs is important, but it cannot be fully understood without accounting for their personal identity, class and heritage. Continuing on from this point, Mendes (2015) considers that it is the impact of culture and religion on the person, and how this influences their personal belief and behaviours, that is arguably more important than learning about differing religions or culture. Here, I argue that knowing about the religious, spiritual and cultural needs of your patient gives you a starting point in which to assess and ask those important questions needed to determine the best course of action for your patient, which is of paramount importance when we are dealing with their health needs, both physical and psychological.

So far, there has been a focus on how religion, spirituality and belief impact on physical health and patients' needs. Next, we will spend some time focusing on mental health and religion, as the emotional and psychological well-being of our patients is as important as their physical well-being. The NMC standards clearly state that promoting and improving 'mental, physical, behavioural and other health related outcomes' is important (NMC, 2018, p12). Also, there is an evidence base that demonstrates a strong link between physical and mental health. Oman and Thoresen (2005) suggest that physical health benefits from religion and can facilitate gains in mental health, such as better social relationships, coping ability and health behaviours. There is a give-and-take relationship between physical and mental health.

Mental health and religion

Is a patient that has mental health issues benefiting from being religious or spiritual? As a healthcare professional who should deliver evidence-based care, this is a vital question. However, the answer to this question is by no means straightforward. First, in diverse communities, which we have discussed in this book, some have a disproportionately higher level of mental health problems compared to the general population:

Learning disability – Between 25 and 40% of people with learning disabilities also experience mental health problems.

(Foundation for People with Learning Disabilities, 2019)

Black Asian minority ethnic (BAME) community – Generally considered to be at increased risk of poor mental health compared to the general white population. If you look at the BAME based on gender women of colour experience mental health issues more so than men.

(Mental Health Foundation, 2016)

People from ethnic minorities are less likely than their White British counterparts to have contacted their general practitioner (GP) about mental health concerns, to be prescribed antidepressants, or to be referred to specialist mental health services.

(Codjoe et al., 2019, p225)

Roma gypsy traveller – In Northern Ireland, the suicide rate among male Irish travellers is 6.6 times higher than that of men in the general population.

(Mental Health Foundation, 2016)

Gay and bisexual men – have higher risks of substance abuse, suicide, depression, and anxiety.

(Lassiter et al., 2017)

Therefore, when caring for patients in diverse communities, it is important that you take into consideration the patient's mental health as well as their physical health. The Mental Health Foundation (2016) also highlighted that some healthcare professionals are less likely to diagnose a mental health condition in BAME groups and that some BAME members are less likely to seek help. These issues are discussed in more detail in Chapter 8.

Participation in religion has been related to a psychological state that has been shown to shield against stress and harmful psychological states. The mechanisms that drive these associations are not very clear (Haney and Rollock, 2018). However, the importance of how religion can provide comfort and help, and give meaning to a person's life, bringing a sense of unity to their experience of the world that can be altered due to severe stress or anxiety, must not be undervalued.

The evidence on the effects of religion and spirituality on mental health is complex. We will look at some of the positive and negative impacts on the mental health of some of the diverse groups previously mentioned, as well as what part religion and spirituality play.

Lassiter et al. (2017) noted the contradictory nature of the evidence around the LGBTQ community, and that religion and spirituality have both positive and negative effects on this community's health. They found that spirituality and religion relate to lower levels of depression, suicide, stress and post-traumatic stress. Religious connection has been found to be associated with positive affect, better quality of life, greater life satisfaction and higher morale. The negative aspects have been that:

religion, particularly negative religious coping (e.g., passive reliance on the sacred; feeling abandoned by the sacred and extrinsic religious orientation) and spirituality, to a lesser extent, have also been associated with poor mental health outcomes.

(Lassiter et al., 2017, p2)

Haney and Rollock (2018) consider what it is about religion that can make it a useful part of managing mental health problems. They suggest the reason for this is the variety of parts involved in many differing religious experiences that offer support to adherents. One aspect is through social interactions that occur when meeting in a place of worship such as a church, synagogue or temple. Hanney and Rollock (2018) also go on to consider the following reasons:

three aspects of religiosity may explain the relationship between religion and the mental health outcomes that it predicts: (a) extrinsic factors, including religious activities and social support from a religious community; (b) intrinsic factors, such as private prayer or the ability to derive meaning from a religious perspective; and (c) religious doubt, the questioning or feeling of disconnection from religious belief that may undermine religious coping and other spiritual processes.

(p2)

The last idea of religious doubt can negatively cause shame or guilt that may cause self-esteem issues or guilt due to having a mental health problem. This may lead to damaging relationships with family friends and healthcare professionals.

Research by Codjoe et al. (2019) shows that BAME service users think that a positive relationship with their religion is essential to wellness and is more important than a medically focused view of mental healthcare. In the black African community in England, the largest concentration of African Christianity outside of Africa can be found in the Borough of Southwark in London (Codjoe et al., 2019). This again highlights the importance of religion in connection to diverse groups and mental health. Codjoe et al. (2019) also go on to state that the Church can be used to reach members of the black African community in a way to highlight that having mental health issues is something that needs addressing, as well as the importance of getting help and using the mental health services available (Turner et al., 2018). Mental health diagnosis such as depression is as important as a physiological diagnosis such as diabetes; both require the appropriate intervention by a healthcare professional.

It is important to make a concentrated effort to appreciate each person for who they are, incorporating their ethnicity, culture, sexual orientation, learning disability, and religious and spiritual needs. As diverse as communities are, recognising the need to respect the diverse meaning systems of each person is vital (Starnino, 2016). In other words, you need to find out how everyone interprets their lives and religious or spiritual needs. As Codjoe et al. (2019) suggest, as mental healthcare professionals (MHCPs) (but valuable to all HCPs), 'sensitivity and understanding of differing cultural and religious beliefs and how these relate to knowledge, attitudes and behaviours towards mental health' is important (p225).

Concept summary: acculturation

The exposure that occurs in parts of the UK due to the diversity of the population can cause a process called acculturation. The exposure of differing cultural groups can influence them to the extent that they adapt their original views, values and beliefs (Nyatanga, 2018). This can also impact on how they interpret their religious beliefs. Such modification (acculturation) suggests that different cultural groups may adapt their original views, values and beliefs following exposure to other cultures. Such exposure takes place in numerous ways and at different times. The education system is seen as the first and most essential transformer of parental-inspired cultural values and belief systems (Celeste et al., 2016; Nyatanga, 2018).

Religion, spirituality and culture have a strong connection (Dein et al., 2012); therefore, this concept is important for two reasons, particularly as we are focusing on groups that are culturally and religiously diverse. The first is that those who have immigrated from their country of birth to the UK may well hold on to cultural and religious beliefs as they would in their country of origin. However, second- or third-generation immigrants who have been more steeped in British culture may have differing belief systems. Landrine and Klonoff (2004) consider this cultural change as follows:

leaving one's indigenous cultural context to spend increasing time in an alternative (e.g., Anglo) one; acculturation refers to the extent to which those who do so (i.e., ethnic minorities) retain their indigenous culture vs. adopt the alternative host (Anglo) culture as a result.

They argue that for minorities, the following could occur:

1. losing behaviours, beliefs, practices, and values specific to their minority culture, and simultaneously, 2. gaining behaviours, beliefs, practices, and values of the Anglo host culture, thereby resulting in four possible outcomes. Ethnic minorities can remain immersed in their indigenous culture (Separated, Traditional), can fully adopt Anglo culture (Acculturated, Assimilated), can be immersed equally in both cultures (Bicultural), or in neither culture (Marginalized).

(p527)

So, what does this all mean for you as a healthcare professional? Being familiar with the religious, spiritual and cultural beliefs of your patient is important. However, just as important is your ability to be aware that your patient's beliefs may not be as fixed to your understanding of that religion or culture due to acculturation. Clarifying the specific needs of your patient and acknowledging their cultural, religious and spiritual needs is something you must do, as your knowledge of their cultural and religious needs may be insufficient to meet their needs.

Death, diversity, culture and nursing

Death is a part of life and is something that you will experience personally and professionally. It is arguably one of the most challenging aspects of being a nurse. We focus so much attention on what we can do to save or prolong life that death can seem a failure. However, death will come to us all. Sometimes there is time to acclimatise to a pending death and other times there is no warning. It is our responsibility and even accountability, as a registered nurse, to assure that all patients take the journey of death in the most dignified and respectful way possible, endeavouring to meet each individual wish of how, when and where death should take place and helping them make varied decisions at the end of life (Phillips et al., 2019). However, communities that share cultural and religious beliefs make sense of death in differing ways: 'Religion, belief and spirituality are conceptual informants of how individuals experience death, dying and bereavement' (Pentaris, 2018, p116).

The South Asian population in the UK continues to be the largest ethnic minority group (ONS, 2012). Venkatasalu (2017) identified that South Asians continue to follow their cultural values and beliefs on death, dying and bereavement, such as wishing to die at home rather than at a hospital or hospice. As with some African cultures, Islamic tradition favours supporting the dying person's family by going to their homes in large numbers and coming together to comfort the immediate family. In Islam, this is considered as Sunna (a practice of the Prophet Muhammad). Do not assume that certain ethnic groups always align with certain religions, because this is not the case. People of varied ethnicities, cultures and nationalities practise Islam, and there are varied types of Islam as there are varied types of Christianity.

Perhaps not surprisingly, nurses are afraid to inform the family about a patient death, preparing the dead patient, performing religious and spiritual practices, and supporting the dead patient's family (Khalaf et al., 2018, p234). What we will do here is one of these areas: informing the family that their loved one has died. To help you with this difficult task of informing the family of a deceased patient on the phone, see Activity 6.2.

Activity 6.2 Communication

Watch the video on delivering the news of a death by telephone by following the below link.

www.sad.scot.nhs.uk/video-wall/

(Continued)

(Continued)

Breaking the news of a death can be particularly challenging for health and social care staff when circumstances require them to do it by telephone. This video aims to help professionals prepare for and undertake these conversations.

The video gives some useful advice on what should be said and how, which can be used for your future practice. As a member of the team, it may be your responsibility to make this call.

In Western society, death can be seen as a failure, and maintaining life for as long as possible is the goal (Wilkins et al., 2010). However, there are multiple and multi-faceted religious viewpoints of the world's religious traditions on the issue of death. When confronting issues on death, religious perspectives can give a framework in which to formulate and grapple with what it is to be human, how death is a part of life, and what happens after death. Even when your patient and you may no longer consider yourself religious because religion is such an integral part of various cultures, it can influence your ideas and beliefs around death (Setta and Shemie, 2015).

In light of the discussion on death, when delivering care to a person at the end of life, being aware of cultural and religious needs of differing communities is important, but, as you will see, determining what is right for the dying person and the people most important to them requires you to ask questions.

End-of-life care in diverse communities

In light of what has been discussed so far, the necessity to capture the needs of cultural, religious and ethnic groups is important. However, those in our communities with specific needs, such as learning disabilities (LD) in palliative care, require special attention. Evidence consistently highlights that the end-of-life needs of patients with LD is a real challenge to provide due to 'disadvantaging issues and circumstances including difficulties with cognition, understanding and communication, complexities in decision-making processes, high levels of co-morbidities and mental health issues, and complex social circumstance' (Tuffrey-Wijne et al., 2016, p447), and this is as unacceptable as patients from other diverse groups. Nyatanga (2018) considers concentrating on the patient as a person rather than as a cultural being, asking questions about what the dying person's wishes are in a sensitive and respectful manner, and what you can do to help them. This may seem obvious, and this should be done for all patients; however, with patients who have a learning disability, that discussion may not be with the patients, but could be with carers, family members or legal guardians. However, do not assume that having an LD means that the patient cannot participate in these important decision-making conversations around end of life (Moro et al., 2017). Adding your own cultural and religious uncertainty and knowledge deficient as a healthcare professional can make these conversations even more challenging.

Some understanding of what is meant by end of life is also needed. You may have considered it means imminent death, but this is not the case. End of life encompasses patients 'approaching the end of life' when they are likely to die within the next 12 months. This includes patients whose death is imminent (expected within a few hours or days) (GMC, 2019). It is vital to support not only the patient, but their family members and significant others, through this particularly sad time, when an advanced, progressive, incurable illness takes hold and the patient and families need support through the last phase of life and into bereavement (NHS Scotland, 2019; NICE, 2017b). The NMC code of conduct states the following:

Make sure that people's physical, social and psychological needs are assessed and responded to. To achieve this, you must: 3.2 recognise and respond compassionately to the needs of those who are in the last few days and hours of life.

(NMC, 2015, p7)

It is our responsibility, as nurses, to work collaboratively with the patient and the family to ensure that death is managed with the utmost dignity and respect, as well as assuring the care needs of our patients are carried out. Different communities have religious, spiritual and cultural needs that should be determined and valued.

Case study

Elliot is a 55-year-old man with Down syndrome and end stage dementia, and is being looked after by his younger sister, Marion, and their father, Albert, at home. The GP knows the family well, as does the district nurse, who is your practice assessor (PA) on your community placement. The GP has reviewed Elliot. His breathing, which became laboured overnight, has been stabilised, and assessment indicates that he has only a few days left to live. The family are understandably upset and want to do the best they can for Elliot. You ask your PA if the family has any specific religious or other needs that have been previously discussed, and it has not as they have not wanted to talk about it when broached with them previously.

What questions could your PA and you ask to best find out this information?

An answer can be found at the end of this chapter, which you may find helpful.

Marion, Elliot's sister, has been going to church over the past six months, and she has found that it has helped her manage her feelings about the worsening condition of her brother. She says that she would talk to her brother about what was said at church and that she felt he gained some comfort from it, and would like to ask the head of her church to come to the house and see Elliot, which perhaps could help all the family deal with her brother dying.

The support that can be given by religious leader has a place in end-of-life care that is valuable, whether that be from your patient or their family members' personal religious leader or organised through us, as nurses. The role of chaplaincy can be key. Chaplaincy is based on Christian traditions, but now Buddhists, imans and rabbis, as well as vicars and priests, can fall under the term 'chaplaincy'. What they have in common is the ability to give religious and spiritual care, compassion, listening and cultural understanding, particularly, but not exclusively, at the end of life and when the patient is dying (Sanford and Michon, 2019). The receiver of chaplaincy support does not need to be of a particular religion. The all-important emotional support that can be given through the chaplaincy service is of significance to the patient and family members (Fitchett, 2017). However, do not think that your patient and their family members may not want to talk to you about their religious and spiritual needs, and that once referred to chaplaincy you do not need to do anything else. Evidence indicates otherwise, and that discussing the religious or spiritual aspects of death, dying and treatment with their healthcare professional is also important; therefore, you need to be prepared for this conversation (Fitchett, 2017). Going back to RCN (2011) guidance on religious and spiritual care can be of help.

Chapter summary

First, it is important to state that many of the points raised here relate to all our patients that we meet daily in a variety of different hospital and community settings. The importance of communication, respect, dignity, and person-centred, individualised care within the context of religion, spirituality, death and end-of-life care cannot be underestimated. All our patients deserve this. We all have differing religious and spiritual beliefs, even when we do not consider ourselves religious, and to some extent this guides us as humans – and nurses.

That being said, the evidence strongly identifies that patients who have learning disabilities and those of differing religions and ethnicities than the predominant white Christian tradition in the UK do not view death and end-of-life issues in the same way, and experience poor care around death and end-of-life care. This is not acceptable, and with the right knowledge and being able to ask the right questions, better clinical decisions can be made with and for the patient in a sensitive and respectful manner. Without this, it will be tough to give the level of care that these and all our patients deserve around such sensitive issues.

Activities: brief outline answers

Activity 6.1   Critical thinking (p116)

Standard 1: Spiritual and religious care

In the standards for NHS Scotland Chaplaincy Services (2007), spiritual and religious care are defined as follows:

> *religious care is given in the context of shared religious beliefs, values, liturgies and lifestyle of a faith community. Spiritual care is usually given in a one to one relationship, is completely person centred and makes no assumptions about personal conviction of life orientation. Spiritual care is not necessarily religious. Religious care, at its best is always spiritual.*

(p3)

Case study (p125)

Nyatanga (2018) gives a comprehensive idea on the types of questions that could be asked and why. Of course, not all need to be asked, and not all at the same time, but you can see that specific questions must be asked to get as much information as possible to assess the needs of your patient and their family and carers.

- What brings you here today?
- What is bothering you the most?
- Could you help me to understand what is worrying you (if you think there could be psychosocial issues) or bothering you (if you suspect physical issues such as pain)?

These questions will allow you to address their concerns (agenda) first by understanding their priorities before you can offer the best support available/possible. Proactive caring involves asking your patient direct questions. For example:

- Do you have any rituals/practices that I should be aware of in order to help you with your illness while you are with us?

Further reading

Burnard, P. and Gill, P. (2014) *Culture, Communication and Nursing.* London: Routledge.

This book provides helpful guidance on how to communicate in an effective and culturally sensitive way.

Chopra, D. (2012) *Spiritual Solutions: Answers to Life's Greatest Challenges.* New York: Harmony.

This book provides advice and tips on how to expand your awareness to help deal with complex situations and challenges.

Useful websites

The Worldwide Hospice Palliative Care Alliance

www.thewhpca.org

An international non-governmental organisation focusing exclusively on hospice and palliative care development worldwide. They are a network of national and regional hospice and palliative care organisations and affiliate organisations.

WHO Key Facts: Palliative Care

www.who.int/news-room/fact-sheets/detail/palliative-care

The World Health Organization addresses key issues relating to palliative care globally, looking at what is being done to improve end-of-life care.

WHO Definition of Palliative Care

www.who.int/cancer/palliative/definition/en/

A definition of palliative care and ways in which to implement palliative care across the life span.

Marie Curie: What Are Palliative Care and End of Life Care?

www.mariecurie.org.uk/help/support/diagnosed/recent-diagnosis/palliative-care-end-of-life-care

Marie Curie is a UK-based charity that focuses on care and support for the terminally ill. This page helps to explain terminology such as palliative care and end-of-life care, and how this type of care can help the terminally ill.

NHS: What End of Life Care Involves

www.nhs.uk/conditions/end-of-life-care/what-it-involves-and-when-it-starts/

This NHS website gives more definitions of terms, as well as what can be done and who can be involved in end-of-life care.

NHS Inform: Palliative Care

www.nhsinform.scot/care-support-and-rights/palliative-care

Palliative care is about improving the quality of life of anyone facing a life-threatening condition. It includes physical, emotional and spiritual care. This is a comprehensive look at symptom control, the conditions that can cause palliative care needs, practical help, planning for the future, and preparing for death and bereavement.

Age UK: End of Life Issues

www.ageuk.org.uk/information-advice/health-wellbeing/relationships-family/end-of-life-issues/

Age UK: Coping with Bereavement

www.ageuk.org.uk/information-advice/health-wellbeing/relationships-family/bereavement/

Both of these Age UK pages are useful in directing patients and their families to information on end-of-life care and coping with bereavement.

NHS Education for Scotland: Support around Death

www.sad.scot.nhs.uk

This NHS Education for Scotland website aims to support healthcare staff who are working with patients, carers and families before, at and after death. It provides key information on the clinical, legislative and practical issues involved.

Chapter 7

Public health
Meeting the needs of diverse communities

Gillian Craig and Caroline McGraw

NMC Standards of Proficiency for Registered Nurses

This chapter will address the following platforms and proficiencies:

Platform 2: Promoting health and preventing ill health

2.2　demonstrate knowledge of epidemiology, demography, genomics and the wider determinants of health, illness and wellbeing and apply this to an understanding of global patterns of health and wellbeing outcomes.

2.3　understand the factors that may lead to inequalities in health outcomes.

2.12　protect health through understanding and applying the principles of infection prevention and control, including communicable disease surveillance and anti-microbial stewardship and resistance.

Platform 5: Leading and managing nursing care and working in teams

5.12　understand the mechanisms that can be used to influence organisational change and public policy, demonstrating the development of political awareness and skills.

Platform 7: Coordinating care

7.4　identify the implications of current health policy and future policy changes for nursing and other professions and understand the impact of policy changes on the delivery and coordination of care.

7.13　demonstrate an understanding of the importance of exercising political awareness throughout their career, to maximise the influence and effect of registered nursing on quality of care, patient safety and cost effectiveness.

Chapter aims

After reading this chapter, you will be able to:

- describe the key principles of a public health approach;
- discuss the needs of diverse communities affected by communicable (e.g. tuberculosis) and non-communicable (e.g. diabetes) diseases and the need for a public health preventative approach;
- appreciate the importance of tackling not only individual factors and health behaviours, but also structural factors, as part of a public health approach; and
- demonstrate an awareness of different policy contexts and how to influence policy to address health inequalities in diverse communities.

Introduction

Public health is defined as 'the art and science of preventing disease, prolonging life and promoting health through the organized efforts of society' (Acheson, 1988, p4).

There is a range of approaches and interventions that aim to prevent disease and improve the health of the public. In this chapter, we discuss interventions at the individual and community level, such as screening and immunisation, and those aimed at the population level, including government legislation. The Soft Drinks Industry Levy (discussed later in the chapter) regulating the quantity of sugar in soft drinks and the ban on smoking in public places are examples of population-level interventions. The introduction of the NHS in 1948 was arguably one of the most significant public health interventions, paid for through taxation, with its principles of care for all regardless of need, and free at the point of access. Interventions can be universal, aimed at the wider population, or targeted at particular groups or communities who are at increased risk.

A public health approach is based on a set of principles, including: the focus on improving the health of the population; a role for government in achieving public health; an emphasis on prevention; the need to address the underlying social determinants of health that cause health inequalities; and, we might argue, the involvement of individuals and communities in the co-production of knowledge about their health and interventions designed to improve health and tackle health inequalities.

The Commission on Social Determinants of Health (WHO, 2008b) (introduced in Chapter 2) highlighted how individual life chances vary dramatically, including illness burden and premature mortality, depending on the circumstances in which people are born, grow, live and age. Differences in life expectancy (discussed in Chapter 2) are particularly marked in diverse communities. We know that people from non-white ethnic groups (e.g. Bangladeshi, Pakistani, Indian and Caribbean groups) experience worse health compared to those from white ethnic groups. Other groups also experience worse health and worse health outcomes compared to the rest of the population. These include those seeking asylum, some vulnerable groups of migrants, people with a learning disability, homeless and prison populations, looked after children, gypsy and traveller communities, sex workers, and those from LGBTQ communities.

In 2014, Public Health England set seven priorities for improving public health: (1) tackling obesity (particularly in children); (2) reducing smoking; (3) reducing harm from alcohol; (4) securing the best start in life for children by tackling the wider determinants of health; (5) preventing the risk of dementia in older people; (6) reducing tuberculosis; and (7) tackling antimicrobial resistance (PHE, 2014d). We have designed our activities in this chapter to reflect these priorities in order to illustrate how nurses can contribute to the public health of diverse communities.

Nurses across different fields of practice will contribute to public health in a variety of ways. The Nursing and Midwifery Council, for example, has developed standards of proficiency for specialist community public health nurses (NMC, 2004). These expect health visitors, school nurses and occupational health nurses to search for health needs through surveillance and assessment of the population's health and well-being, including the analysis of data, identifying risk and screening for disease. Nurses will create awareness of health needs in terms of the actions individuals and groups can take to improve their health and well-being. Nurses will be expected to appraise and influence policies affecting health and make recommendations for change to improve health and well-being. Finally, nurses will facilitate health-enhancing activities that promote and protect the population's health and well-being. They will be expected to apply leadership skills to manage people, projects and resources to improve health and well-being.

In order to illustrate how some groups experience particular health risks and potentially worse health outcomes compared to the general population, we have selected a number of scenarios to illustrate health need in diverse communities and the corresponding public health approaches that nurses can adopt, such as:

- addressing the wider determinants of health through collaborative care packages for young people with tuberculosis who are seeking asylum;
- using local authority health profiles to explore inequalities in smoking, physical activity and alcohol-related harm in England in the context of deprivation and ethnicity;
- protecting the health of homeless people by improving the uptake of influenza immunisation;
- preventing premature mortality through cancer screening in black men and women with a learning disability; and
- action on smoking in the LGBTQ community.

There is a tendency to blame individuals for their poor health or assume that poor health can be corrected through education and the provision of information, rather than addressing the underlying social determinants that cause ill health and influence health choices. In order to counter this, we highlight the role of both structural factors (e.g. the cost of healthcare, where this is not freely available) and what might be viewed as a suboptimal response of the health services (e.g. poor care, lack of integration of health and social care, low practitioner awareness of risk in relation to culture and diversity, health promotion policies that fail to reach diverse communities). In addition to individual and biological differences, these factors also contribute to the poor health that some groups experience.

First, we will explore the transition from communicable diseases as a major cause of death in the nineteenth century to non-communicable diseases (NCDs) as the major cause of preventable deaths in contemporary industrialised countries as a rationale for the need for public health prevention and your role as a nurse in promoting public health. We will look at different policies underpinning nursing practice and how you can address inequalities by influencing policy in order to achieve good health for individuals, families and communities.

Scenario: Changes in the causes of death in East London

Annie was born in Stepney in November 1874. She was the youngest of five children born to Thomas and Margaret. Thomas worked as a coal porter and Margaret as a sack maker. The family shared a one-room dwelling. Annie died aged just 13 months. The cause of death was recorded as tuberculosis. Her death was registered by her father, who went on to register the deaths of Annie's twin brothers from the same cause the following year.

Florence was born in Poplar in November 1948. She and her two sisters were the first generation of children in her family to all survive into adulthood. On leaving school aged 15 years, Florence worked at a local sugar refinery. She was diagnosed with chronic obstructive pulmonary disease (COPD) aged 55 and Type 2 diabetes aged 58. Ill health forced Florence to retire in 1996. Her retirement was marked by repeated acute exacerbations of COPD and hyperglycaemia. She was admitted to hospital on her seventieth birthday with community-acquired pneumonia. She died three days later. Florence was survived by her two sisters.

Changing patterns of disease and a changing demography in the UK

In nineteenth-century Britain, infectious diseases such as tuberculosis were the leading cause of death, particularly in young children. Low life expectancy was due to the high rates of infant mortality. In 1841, a young baby girl would not expect to reach her 43rd birthday, compared to a life expectancy of 82.8 years in 2011 (ONS, 2015).

These changes can be explained by improvements in public health measures, including sanitation, the introduction of safe drinking water, improvements in housing, better diet, and childhood immunisation. As life expectancy has increased, new threats in the form of NCDs (such as cancer, stroke and heart disease) have taken over as the leading causes of death in older age groups rather than children (Fenton, 2016).

The UK has undergone significant demographic changes over the last century. Not only has the size of the population grown from 27 million in 1850 to 66 million in 2017, but black and ethnic minority groups now comprise 12.9 per cent of the population and there are approximately 9.4 million migrants (ONS, 2018). The population is also ageing, with 18.2 per cent aged over 65. In 2016, just over 1 million people identified as lesbian, gay or bisexual, representing 2 per cent of the population (ONS, 2016). The Foundation for People with Learning Disabilities (2019) report that 1.5 million people are living with a learning disability. Approximately 58,000 people living in England and Wales identified themselves as gypsy or Irish traveller in the 2011 census (ONS, 2014), and 1 in every 200 people in the UK are homeless (Shelter, 2017).

Although people may be living longer, it is estimated that 15 million in England are living with a long-term condition such as diabetes or COPD (Department of Health, 2012b). The different health patterns of diverse communities, as well as their specific health and social care needs, will require nurses to have specialist skills and approaches to tackling health and social inequality given these groups are often underserved by mainstream services.

Underserved populations and inclusion health

Public Health England highlights the importance of language in defining underserved populations who do not access mainstream services:

> *People in this population have previously been described as 'hard-to-reach': this description can imply an active withdrawal of people from services but the lived experience of many is that services simply do not map to their needs in terms of accessibility, acceptability or suitability. 'Under-served' more accurately describes the experience of the population and puts the onus on service commissioners and providers to design and deliver services appropriate to the needs of the population.*

(PHE, 2017d, p6)

In recognition that groups may be underserved, a new field of practice has emerged called inclusion health. Inclusion health has been defined as 'a service, research, and policy agenda that aims to prevent and redress health and social inequities among the most vulnerable and excluded populations' (Luchenski et al., 2018, p266). Public health approaches that aim to redress social exclusion are discussed in the scenarios later in this chapter.

The changing epidemiology of disease: from communicable to non-communicable diseases

Epidemiology is the study of the number of people affected by a disease. The World Health Organization defines epidemiology as 'the study of the distribution and determinants of health-related states or events (including disease), and the application of this study to the control of diseases and other health problems' (WHO, n.d. a). Epidemiology can tell us about population health, morbidity and mortality. It can provide data highlighting groups at greater risk of ill health or social issues such as homelessness. It can provide us with information about trends (e.g. whether a health or social issue is improving or getting worse over time). This can be useful in terms of measuring the impact of interventions, such as the introduction of Streptomycin (chemotherapy) for the treatment of tuberculosis (TB) and immunisation (BCG) for the prevention of TB (see Figure 7.1).

We will now consider the changing epidemiology of tuberculosis and diabetes. We have chosen these examples to demonstrate the transition of the disease burden from communicable to non-communicable diseases over time and because particular communities are disproportionately affected by these diseases and are at risk of poorer health outcomes compared to the general population. For example, TB no longer affects the general population, but targets vulnerable groups, such as homeless people, who are often underserved. Groups at particular risk of diabetes include people from South Asia and other black and minority ethnic groups.

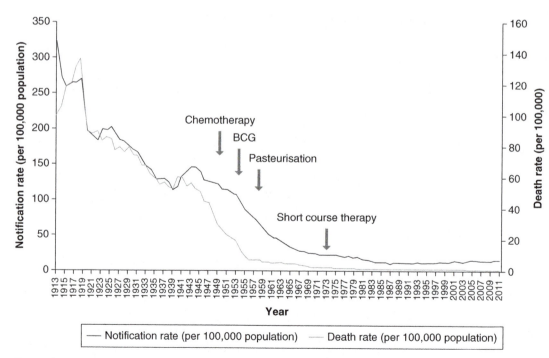

Figure 7.1   Notification rates and death rates, England and Wales, 1913–2011

Source: Statutory notifications of infectious diseases (NOIDS), ONS mid-year population estimates (HPA, 2013)

Tuberculosis: an example of a communicable disease

Tuberculosis is an infectious bacterial disease that can affect any part of the body, including the skeleton, organs, lymph glands and lungs (pulmonary TB). Only when it affects the lungs can it be passed on from person to person, through coughing or sneezing. Symptoms of TB include a persistent cough, loss of appetite, weight loss and fever (night sweats). Without treatment, it can cause serious morbidity and mortality. People living with TB are also stigmatised (see Chapter 2 and the additional resources at the end of this chapter), which may deter them from seeking healthcare or affect their ability to follow their treatment plan.

The number of people reported to have TB in 1913 in England and Wales was 120,000, compared to 5,102 people in 2017 (PHE, 2017d). Figure 7.1 demonstrates the decline in the number of people diagnosed with TB before the introduction of chemotherapy in the 1940s. Prior to this, people with TB were segregated and cared for in sanatoria, with bed rest and fresh air the main form of treatment. The decline in the incidence of TB (the number of new cases in any given period) coincided with public health sanitary measures, slum clearance, improvements in housing, and better standards of living more generally (Gandy, 2003). Living in poor-quality and overcrowded housing was, and continues to be, a risk factor for TB and transmission of the disease. Further decreases in the rate of TB were witnessed following the introduction of the BCG vaccination in secondary schools in the 1950s.

Whereas in the nineteenth century TB affected the general population, in contemporary Britain it mainly affects those experiencing deprivation. For example, epidemiological data demonstrate that people living in the top 10 per cent most deprived communities are seven times more likely to be at risk of TB compared with the least deprived, and people born outside the country are 13 times more likely to be at risk (PHE, 2017d). Not all migrants have the same risk, however, and it can depend on patterns of migration and how common TB is in the country where someone was exposed to the disease. Moreover, underserved populations are twice as likely to develop drug-resistant TB, to not complete their treatment, and to die of the disease (PHE, 2017d). Although the number of new cases of people living with TB is declining overall, the number of people with social risk factors, such as homelessness, contact with the criminal justice system, and alcohol and substance misuse, is increasing. These social risk factors can be a reason why these populations are underserved. People who also have diabetes or HIV (both risk factors for TB) may experience more complex health issues that can affect treatment outcomes.

TB in underserved populations presents particular challenges for the healthcare sector as these groups also experience additional health and social care needs (see case study on pages 140–1). They often require additional support with their TB care in order to complete a course of antibiotics, involving several months of treatment, and there is increasing acknowledgement of the need to address the adverse social issues faced by such groups (such as lack of housing and destitution) that may prevent them from prioritising their health and adhering to care plans.

Moreover, traditional models of healthcare delivery cannot always reach these groups (PHE, 2017d). Research has identified unexpectedly high rates of mortality for those co-infected with HIV in the UK, attributed to late diagnosis of TB and the start of their treatment (Zenner et al., 2015). Nearly one-third of people with pulmonary TB experienced a delay of four months between the onset of their symptoms and receiving treatment in 2017, and delays were most marked in those aged over 65 (PHE, 2017d).

Delays are attributed to both patient and provider behaviour. For example, a GP may fail to recognise the symptoms of TB. People may confuse their symptoms with other illness (such as the common cold or alcohol or drug misuse) and not seek healthcare. Similarly, a person may not work in occupations that allow time off work to attend medical appointments or that pay sickness benefits. Furthermore, people may fear a diagnosis of TB because of the stigma associated with it. Campaigns that raise awareness of symptoms, as well as how to access care and counter the effects of stigma and discrimination, are important components of a public health approach to reducing and treating TB (see resource at the end of the chapter).

Addressing TB in underserved populations is a key area for action (PHE, 2015a, 2017d). Mobile X-ray screening units, which can outreach service to hostels, prisons and a range of community settings, as well as the role of support workers and community agencies, are increasingly recognised as an integral and cost-effective aspect of TB care. Equity of access to care, clear pathways to diagnosis, and enhanced case management to address social risk factors are also key elements of the public health approach. The importance of developing collaborative health and social care packages of support that address the social determinants of health and enable people with TB to prioritise their health is illustrated in the case study on pages 140–1.

TB remains one of the major causes of death globally, particularly of women and children and people living with HIV/AIDS. In 2016, 10.4 million people were sick with TB and it was responsible for 1.7 million deaths worldwide (WHO, 2018b). The argument for the need to address TB in the global context, if we wish to tackle TB in the UK, is compelling.

Diabetes: an example of a non-communicable disease

Approximately 41 million deaths globally are attributable to NCDs that are largely preventable, cardiovascular diseases, cancer, respiratory diseases (e.g. COPD) and diabetes being the most common causes (WHO, 2018a). Tobacco use, unhealthy diet, physical inactivity and harmful use of alcohol increase the risk of NCDs.

We provide an exercise later in the chapter that allows you to identify behavioural risk factors in the local authority where you work or live (see Activity 7.1).

Type 2 diabetes (T2D) is an increasing public health problem and accounts for 90 per cent of diabetes cases globally (Candler et al., 2018). In the UK, the prevalence of diabetes (i.e. the number of people in the population living with diabetes) in primary care doubled from 2.60 in 2001 to 5.32 in 2013 (see Table 7.1). These rates are similar to other European countries (such as Denmark and Sweden) but lower than those in Russia and the United States (International Diabetes Federation, 2017).

Year	%
2001	2.60
2003	3.11
2005	3.66
2007	4.10
2009	4.56
2011	4.98
2013	5.32

Table 7.1 Increases in diabetes prevalence in primary care

Source: Sharma et al. (2016)

The burden of diabetes is not equitably distributed across society. Black and minority ethnic groups in high-income countries such as the US and the UK are disproportionally affected. For example, in the US, diabetes is more likely to affect Native Americans, non-Hispanic black, Hispanic, and Asian American populations (Centers for Disease Control and Prevention, 2011). In the UK, diabetes disproportionally affects black and South Asian communities. The percentage of doctor-diagnosed diabetes is almost double in the Bangladeshi male community compared to the general population (see Table 7.2). The statistics presented here are taken from the Health Survey for England

Ethnic group	Men (%)	Women (%)
Bangladeshi	8.2	5.2
Black African	5	2.1
Black Caribbean	10	8.4
Chinese	3.8	3.3
Indian	10.1	5.9
Irish	3.6	2.3
Pakistani	7.3	8.6
General population	4.3	3.4

Table 7.2 Prevalence of doctor-diagnosed diabetes (Type 1 and Type 2) in adults by ethnic group

Source: NHS Health and Social Care Information Centre (2005)

2004 (NHS Health and Social Care Information Centre, 2005). While more recent health surveys have been conducted, no data have been made available to describe the prevalence of diabetes in different communities.

Diabetes is associated with microvascular and macrovascular complications. Microvascular complications are caused by damage to small blood vessels, and include diabetic retinopathy, nephropathy and neuropathy. Macrovascular complications include cardiovascular disease. Ethnic differences exist in the epidemiology of these complications. For example, in one study of T2D, the prevalence of diabetic retinopathy was 38 per cent in white Europeans compared to 52.4 per cent in African/African Caribbean communities and 43 per cent in South Asian communities (Sivaprasad et al., 2012). By way of contrast, there was evidence of less neuropathy in people from Indian Asian backgrounds with T2D, leading to lower levels of diabetic foot ulceration in this population (Abbott et al., 2010).

There are multiple factors that contribute to ethnic disparities in diabetes. At the individual level, these include biological factors, health behaviours and early life events (Golden et al., 2012). Biological factors relate to differences in fat distribution, glucose metabolism, insulin resistance and glycaemic control in different ethnic groups. Health behaviours include differences in physical activity, smoking and self-monitoring of blood glucose. Early life events include prenatal undernutrition, maternal stress and maternal obesity during pregnancy. These early life events highlight the importance of policies and interventions across the life course, including perinatal and maternal health, from conception to the first two years of life and beyond.

While individual differences may go some way to accounting for the variations in diabetes prevalence and health outcomes, for people with diabetes the contribution of the wider social and structural determinants need to be considered. A survey of barriers to people with diabetes accessing eye care services in eight countries identified cost, long waiting times for appointments, and length of wait in clinics once an appointment had been scheduled (DR Barometer, n.d.). Proximity to care was also a factor. Few people were enrolled on diabetes management programmes because they were either not available or people did not know about them. Overcoming these barriers is important given the growing consensus that diabetic retinopathy is preventable through appropriate screening and timely treatment.

Culturally tailored diabetes prevention programmes are also recommended to ensure health messaging campaigns and healthcare interventions are appropriately designed for diverse communities to access them (Lagisetty et al., 2017). Barriers to access to prevention programmes, as well as how to tailor these to the needs of diverse groups, are discussed later in the chapter.

Affordability, in countries that lack universal healthcare, is a significant barrier to tackling health inequalities. For example, in the US, many black and minority ethnic groups lack health insurance, affecting their ability to access healthcare (Spanakis and Golden, 2013).

From evidence to action: the role of the nurse in addressing health inequalities through the Public Health Outcomes Framework (PHOF)

In Chapter 2, you were introduced to the Marmot Review (Marmot et al., 2010). To recap, the Marmot Review recommended an evidence-based strategy to address health inequalities based on six policy objectives. These policy objectives recommended: giving every child the best start in life; enabling children, young people and adults to maximise their capabilities and have control over their lives; creating fair employment and good work opportunities for everyone; ensuring a healthy standard of living for all; creating and developing healthy and sustainable places and communities; and strengthening the role and impact of ill health prevention.

The importance of giving every child the best start in life is because disadvantage – and advantage – are cumulative across the life course, resulting in sustained inequalities that can have effects across generations. Failure to intervene early can have consequences in adult life. For example, approximately 40 per cent of people with a learning disability are not identified in childhood, and people with a learning disability are more likely to end up in custody than the general public (Rickard and Donkin, 2018). They are at increased risk of poor mental health, and it has been estimated that half of the increased risk can be attributed to poverty, poor housing, bullying and discrimination (Rickard and Donkin, 2018).

The Marmot policy objectives broadly inform the Public Health Outcomes Framework (PHOF). Introduced in 2012, the PHOF provides data on a set of health and social indicators, known as the Marmot indicators, which help monitor improvements as a result of public health interventions. They are updated every three years. The purpose of the framework is to increase healthy life expectancy and reduce differences in life expectancy and healthy life expectancy (i.e. not only how long people live, but how well they live). The role of the nurse is to work with other key stakeholders to improve and protect public health. The indicators fall into four domains:

1. addressing the wider determinants of health;

2. health improvement;

3. health protection; and

4. healthcare, public health and preventing premature mortality.

To illustrate the role of the nurse, we have chosen four nursing interventions pertaining to the PHOF and diverse communities.

Domain 1: addressing the wider determinants of health through collaborative care packages for young people with tuberculosis who are seeking asylum

Chapter 2 introduced the role of the wider determinants of health on health inequalities (e.g. income and employment). Although in the UK TB care is free, people who do not have stable housing, access to food, and income may find it difficult to prioritise their health and adhere to their care plans. This will require nurses to work with agencies in the community to develop collaborative care networks that can address these issues with packages of support. This will enable people to successfully complete their treatment. If people stop taking their medication, they can develop more serious forms of drug-resistant TB that are harder and more costly to treat and can have serious implications for individual and community health.

Case study: Collaborative TB care for underserved populations

Faduma was 17 when she started treatment for tuberculosis (six months of antibiotics). She came to England from Somalia seeking asylum aged 9 and was looked after by her older sister. Aged 14, she became homeless following a breakdown in the family relationship. As she was not entitled to housing or benefits because of her immigration status (she had never applied for indefinite leave to remain in her own right), she was left destitute. She relied on friends to house her (sofa-surfing). Faduma was subjected to sexual exploitation and abuse by men. She had been to several organisations seeking assistance but had become mistrustful and disillusioned with the services.

Faduma found it difficult to take her TB medication due to her housing and financial situation. Having nowhere to live, she relied on fast food, which was expensive. Sometimes she missed her medication because where she slept was not where she had left her belongings, including her medication. She stopped taking her medication and failed to attend her clinic appointments. The TB nurse conducted a risk assessment and referred Faduma to a social worker based in the TB clinic for additional support. They developed a joint care plan that catered for both her health and social care needs. After much encouragement and reassurance from the TB team, Faduma began attending her appointments. The nurse and social worker referred Faduma to a local refugee agency for immigration advice. The refugee advisor then made a referral to social services for housing, with supporting evidence from the TB team. The refugee agency also referred Faduma to a solicitor to apply for refugee status and made an application for indefinite leave to remain.

Legal advisors also became involved in Faduma's case following social services' initial reluctance to accept a duty of care for her. Social services later secured housing on a temporary basis in bed and breakfast accommodation, but Faduma once again became at risk of sexual exploitation. Due to a deterioration in her health, and given she was vulnerable and still technically homeless, Faduma was admitted to hospital until appropriate temporary accommodation with support from a care worker could be found. Faduma was granted full refugee status, which entitled her to permanent housing and benefits, and she completed her treatment. This example illustrates the need for social care packages of support in enabling vulnerable people to adhere to their care plans and be cured of TB.

Note: This case study was based on the findings of a research study and adapted for the purpose of this chapter. For more information, see Craig et al. (2008).

Domain 2: using local authority health profiles to explore areas for health improvement

'Health improvement' is a term used to describe interventions that encourage healthy lifestyle choices. Public health profiles of local authorities have been developed by PHE and are designed to provide information about a range of health indicators (e.g. inequalities in alcohol-related harm, smoking, physical activity). They also give information on the percentage of people affected from ethnic minority groups and younger and older age groups. Data in the profiles are benchmarked against the England average. You can compare how the borough you live or work in compares with the rest of England on specific health indicators in Activity 7.1.

Activity 7.1   Evidence-based practice and research

In order to explore areas for health improvement, you will need to look at specific health needs in your area. You can find out about the health of people in local authorities by accessing their online health profiles (see the PHE Health Profile Tool in the useful websites section at the end of the chapter). Choose a local authority and identify the rates of smoking, physical activity and alcohol-related harm in that area. Then check to see if these indicators are significantly worse, no different or significantly better

(Continued)

(Continued)

than the England average. What does the profile tell you about local levels of deprivation, the age profile of the borough and the ethnic composition of the borough? How will deprivation, age and ethnic composition influence your choice of a health improvement intervention?

An outline answer is provided at the end of the chapter.

We will now look at how nurses can protect the health of vulnerable populations.

Domain 3: protecting the health of homeless people by improving the uptake of influenza immunisation

Health protection aims to protect the population from threats, including infectious diseases (e.g. influenza and measles), antibiotic resistance, and radiation and environmental hazards (e.g. air pollution). One key health protection issue is seasonal influenza, an acute respiratory infection caused by the influenza virus. All age groups can be affected, but there are some groups more at risk than others, including pregnant women, older people, people with a long-term condition, and people with compromised immunity (e.g. those with HIV or diabetes).

Lesser-recognised groups at risk of influenza include the homeless and prison populations. These groups are at greater risk of contracting influenza due to higher levels of exposure than the general population, attributed to living in overcrowded settings. They are also at greater risk of serious illness due to the higher prevalence of respiratory illness (e.g. asthma), immunosuppression and other long-term conditions (e.g. cardiovascular disease, diabetes, liver disease) than the general population (Story et al., 2014).

Vaccination is the most effective measure to prevent severe disease caused by influenza. However, uptake rates are lower in the homeless population than in the general population. For example, during 2011–2012, uptake in homeless 16–64-year-olds with a clinical risk factor was 23.7 per cent, compared to national levels of 53.2 per cent, and uptake in homeless people aged over 65 years was 42.9 per cent, compared with 74 per cent nationally (Story et al., 2014). Similarly, uptake rates are currently lower in prison populations than the general population (PHE, 2017b).

Now complete Activity 7.2, which asks you to think about the reasons for differential uptake of immunisation in homeless populations.

Activity 7.2   Critical thinking

As a student, you have a placement with the health inclusion team, a nurse-led community team that provides primary healthcare services for vulnerable groups (including homeless people, refugees, asylum seekers, and drug and alcohol users). The team provides a range of free and confidential services, including a homelessness health check. This check is conducted using the Health Assessment Tool for use by community nurses with people who are homeless (Queens Nursing Institute, 2015). One of the domains covered by the tool is immunisation. An audit has revealed lower levels of seasonal influenza vaccination among people who sleep outside (rough sleepers) compared to people living in temporary accommodation. What are the reasons for this disparity, and how might it be addressed?

An outline answer is provided at the end of the chapter.

Domain 4: preventing premature mortality through cancer screening in black men and women with a learning disability

Health inequalities were discussed in Chapter 2. Groups that experience poor health outcomes and premature mortality are those that are more likely to be socially excluded or underserved. Two examples of where premature mortality can be prevented in diverse communities include screening for prostate cancer in black men and screening for cervical cancer in women with a learning disability.

Prostate cancer screening and black men

Prostate cancer is the most common cancer in the UK, affecting one in eight men, with an increased risk of one in four for those men from a black African or black Caribbean community (Prostate Cancer UK, 2014). Other risk factors include age (over 50 years) and having an immediate male relative with prostate cancer (father or a brother). There is also evidence to suggest that black men have worse survival rates than white men.

There is currently no national screening programme for prostate cancer in the UK. Instead, there is an informed choice programme, called prostate cancer risk management, which relies on individuals requesting a prostate-specific antigen (PSA) test from their GP. However, this approach requires a high degree of prostate cancer awareness. The reason there is no national screening programme is because of concerns regarding the reliability of PSA testing in detecting cancer.

The reasons for ethnic differences in prostate cancer incidence and survival rates are unknown, but are likely to include genetic and biological factors and complex behavioural and socio-economic factors (Jones and Chinegwundoh, 2014). Service provider awareness and behaviour is also a factor. For example, research in the US has reported significant differences in rates of radiation and surgical treatment for prostate cancer between white and black men, with most healthcare services favouring white men (Friedlander et al., 2018). Similarly, in the UK, there is anecdotal evidence that GPs have refused PSA testing or neglected digital rectal examinations in black men despite their elevated risk (Knight, 2012).

To combat prostate cancer, further work is required to ensure that awareness in communities at risk and among healthcare professionals is addressed. In the UK, black men are taking the lead on raising awareness in their communities. For example, the Errol McKellar Foundation was set up by a former Hackney mechanic and Leyton Orient youth team coach who was diagnosed with aggressive prostate cancer in 2010. His mission is to try to talk to as many men as possible to ensure that they are fully aware of the dangers posed by prostate cancer, its potential symptoms, and the tests available (for further information, see the Errol McKellar Foundation website link at the end of this chapter). This example illustrates the power of service users in raising awareness in communities underserved by the formal healthcare sector and the need for nurses to work in partnership with local service users and their carers.

From a practitioner perspective, it is important that nurses (e.g. practice nurses) monitor their unconscious bias (i.e. stereotypes or prejudices about certain group characteristics that individuals form outside their own conscious awareness) when responding to patients requesting PSA testing. One approach would be to audit nursing practice against a set of standards such as those set out in the consensus statement by Prostate Cancer UK (2016).

Cervical cancer screening and women with a learning disability

People with a learning disability experience premature death and die 15 to 20 years earlier than their non-disabled peers. More than a third of these deaths could be prevented with appropriate intervention (HQIP, 2017). In response to the high mortality rates, the national Learning Disabilities Mortality Review was set up in 2015. The programme aims to identify factors contributing to preventable deaths and make recommendations for improving the standard and quality of healthcare. People with a learning disability, as well as their families and carers, have all been involved in developing the programme (HQIP, 2017).

All women and people with a cervix (e.g. some trans men) aged over 25 are entitled to cervical screening every three years. The introduction of screening has halved the incidence of cervical cancer in the UK (Kmietowicz, 2009). However, research suggests that women with a learning disability are less likely to receive screening for cervical cancer compared to the general population (Reynolds et al., 2008). Other neglected groups include LGBTQ people. The low take-up of cervical screening may, in part, be attributable to incorrect information that transmen and lesbian women do not need screening because of their sexual orientation rather than their sexual health needs (LGBT Foundation, 2018). Activity 7.3 invites you to consider how nurses can prevent premature mortality through screening for cervical cancer in women with a learning disability.

Activity 7.3   Communication

You are on placement with a practice nurse. A young woman with a learning disability, aged 26, attends the practice with an eye infection. The practice nurse notices that she has never had cervical screening. Read the guidance by Public Health England on supporting women with a learning disability to access cervical screening (PHE, 2017c) and give your practice supervisor a summary of best practice (see guidance for cervical cancer screening for women with a learning disability at the end of chapter).

As this activity will draw upon your own responses, there is no outline answer provided at the end of this chapter, but guidance is available.

Legislation and public health: should governments intervene in the health of the population?

Criticism of government intervention into the nation's health is often heard with the pejorative term 'nanny state'. Baggott (2011) describes two contrasting political positions on the involvement of government in health matters: liberal-individualistic, which seeks to promote individual liberty and choice, free from state involvement; and collectivist, which sees a role for the state in protecting individuals. Critics of the liberal-individualistic approach argue that government intervention is necessary because people's choices are constrained by factors such as poverty and discrimination. Caraher et al. (2014) provide an example of how access to healthy food choices can be constrained by obesogenic environments (i.e. environments that contribute to obesity), which, they argue, only promote unhealthy choices. Given that unhealthy food is often cheaper than healthy food, as well as the preponderance of fast-food outlets available 24 hours a day, there is increasing availability and opportunity for unhealthy food choices.

There have been calls for mandatory regulation of the food industry to reduce salt and sugar content in food and drink to curb obesity and diabetes (Caraher and Perry, 2017). In April 2018, the government introduced the Soft Drinks Industry Levy (branded the sugar tax) as a key milestone in tackling obesity. Manufacturers are required to reduce the amount of sugar in soft drinks or pay a levy. Companies will be required to pay 24p per litre of drink if it contains 8 grams of sugar per 100 millilitres and 18p per litre of drink if it contains between 5 and 8 grams of sugar per 100 millilitres (HM Treasury, 2015). The legislation is not without controversy, with some arguing this represents a tax on the poor, while others suggest that poorer people are more likely to experience health benefits (Briggs et al., 2013).

Health policy and diverse communities

The importance of the need for good health policy in tackling health inequalities is aptly described by the Commission on Social Determinants of Health:

> *[The] toxic combination of bad policies, economics, and politics is, in large measure responsible for the fact that a majority of people in the world do not enjoy the good health that is biologically possible.*

> (WHO, 2008a, p26)

This would support the view of a strong role for government in improving health and preventing ill health through appropriate economic and political systems and policies that address inequalities.

Politics can be defined as 'the process of influencing the allocation of scarce resources' (Chaffee et al., 2012, p5). McCullough (2014) quotes Shrock (1977) who argues that nurses should develop political awareness 'to understand and analyse the socioeconomic and political background to the services of which they are part, as a potentially powerful group of health care workers'.

Health policy:

> *refers to decisions, plans, and actions that are undertaken to achieve specific health care goals within a society. An explicit health policy can achieve several things: it defines a vision for the future which in turn helps to establish targets and points of reference for the short and medium term. It outlines priorities and the expected roles of different groups and it builds consensus and informs people.*

> (WHO, n.d. b)

Governments introduce policies to address specific problems, and policies change over time due to political, social, economic and cultural developments. Solutions to the problems the policy is trying to address also change over time. Abuse in older people, for example, is increasingly recognised as an issue, perhaps because of people living longer, as well as high-profile cases about abuse of trust by carers and changing attitudes towards older people. Policy does not exist in a vacuum, however, and

Five Year Forward View (NHS England, 2014b)	Set out a vision for how the health service in England should change over the next five years to close the widening gaps in the health of the population, the quality of care and the funding of services.
Five Year Forward View for Mental Health (NHS England, 2016a)	Profiled the current state of mental health service provision in England and made recommendations for better, more responsive and accessible mental health services.
Collaborative TB Strategy for England: 2015 to 2020 (PHE, 2015a)	Outlined how government intended to organise and resource services to tackle TB and identified ten key areas for action, including underserved populations.
Prime Minister's Challenge on Dementia 2020 (Department of Health, 2015b)	Set out a vision to ensure England is the best country in the world for dementia care and support, and for people with dementia, as well as their carers and families, to live.
Childhood Obesity: A Plan for Action (HM Government, 2016a)	Committed to introducing mechanisms to significantly reduce England's rate of childhood obesity, including introducing a Soft Drinks Industry Levy, supporting innovation to help businesses to make their products healthier, and making healthy options available in the public sector.
Action for Diabetes (NHS England, 2014a)	Outlined what action should be undertaken to improve outcomes for people with and at risk of diabetes in England.
Ending Violence against Women and Girls: Strategy 2016–2020 (HM Government, 2016b)	Set out a vision to reduce the prevalence of all forms of violence against women and girls, matched by increases in reporting, police referrals, prosecution and convictions.
A Connected Society: A Strategy for Tackling Loneliness – Laying the Foundations for Change (HM Government, 2018)	A strategy that establishes a foundation to provide opportunities for people to have meaningful contact. GPs in England will be able to refer people experiencing loneliness to community activities.

Table 7.3   Examples of policies guiding public health practice

an understanding of the drivers of policy and the political and economic landscape in which nurses are required to implement policy, as part of their practice, is an important aspect of public health. Table 7.3 outlines some policies influencing nursing practice in England.

The drivers of contemporary policy

The factors that drive the need for policy may include:

- evidence of health need (increases in rates of obesity, smoking, dementia, falls in older people, poor uptake of immunisation, etc.);
- changing societal attitudes and public opinion (e.g. concerns about violence, child health and the need to protect vulnerable groups, and concerns about poverty and the impact on children's health and development);

- pressure groups demanding change and influencing policy, including healthcare professionals, the public, parents, professional bodies, trade unions and voluntary organisations;
- economic costs of disease or welfare (costs to government for treating diseases and the austerity agenda);
- recognition that current practice/service delivery is not fit for purpose and that change needs to be implemented (e.g. the Francis Report (Department of Health, 2013) into the failings of the Mid-Staffordshire NHS Foundation Trust, which recommended the need to develop standards of care);
- evidence reviews (e.g. the Marmot Review on health inequalities); and
- ideology informed by the political positions of different governments (the referendum on leaving the European Union ('Brexit') was not based on evidence, but political ideas).

Influencing policy and decision-making to change health systems and tackle inequalities

Acting to bring about change in policies addressing poverty and inequality is a matter of social justice because some groups experience poorer health outcomes than others and are more adversely affected by policies. There is some evidence to suggest that women, minorities and disabled people were worst hit by the impact of austerity measures implemented by the Conservative–Liberal Democrat Coalition Government (2010–2015), as were more deprived local authorities (Hastings et al., 2013).

The Royal College of Nursing also acknowledges that policy and knowledge development is a defining characteristic of the nursing role (RCN, 2003). Moreover, as nurses act as advocates for their clients/patients, they need to understand how to influence policy to protect vulnerable communities who may be adversely affected by policies. For example, the removal of the spare room subsidy under the Welfare Reform Act 2012, also known as the 'bedroom tax', restricted benefits to people based on their household size rather than their needs. This resulted in a loss of income for some families and disproportionately impacted people with disabilities and long-term conditions (Moffatt et al., 2016).

It has been suggested that nurses do not engage with the policy process due to a perceived lack of 'time and resources, lack of status and decision making power and a possible lack of politicisation of nurses' (Gleeson et al., 2015, p40). However, there are a range of ways that nurses can influence policy, including through membership of a trade union (e.g. UNITE) or professional organisation such as the RCN; by contributing to government (national or local) consultation documents (e.g. on proposed changes to the NHS, legislation regulating sugar and salt content in food, regulation of healthcare professions); by writing to their MP or local councillor about an issue; and by voting in the general and local elections. We provide an activity that would allow you to advocate on behalf of communities by writing to your MP (see Activity 7.4).

Leadership and management

There is evidence that legislation banning smoking in indoor public spaces in England in 2007 has been effective in reducing the number of people who smoke, reducing exposure to second-hand smoke, and reducing the number of hospital admissions for myocardial infarction (Bauld, 2011).

Vulnerable groups may have difficulties accessing smoking cessation programmes, and although they may experience barriers that are common to other groups, they also experience specific barriers (Twyman et al., 2014), which has implications for the content, design and delivery of smoking cessation programmes. Twyman et al. (2014) argue for the need for smoking cessation programmes aimed at the individual, community and social network levels when working with vulnerable groups.

LGBTQ people are more likely to smoke. They are also more likely to experience social disadvantage (e.g. they are more likely to be homeless, experience mental health problems and use drugs) (ODPHP, n.d.). Smoking may be associated with particular lifestyles or used as a coping mechanism. Hence, tackling the underlying reasons for smoking and identifying alternative coping mechanisms will be needed. LGBTQ people may not feel comfortable accessing mainstream services for fear of discrimination. Advice on developing smoking cessation resources for LGBTQ groups are available from the National LGB&T Partnership (see the useful websites section at the end of the chapter). Activity 7.4 invites you to advocate on behalf of an LGBTQ group in relation to tobacco promotion.

Activity 7.4 Influencing policy

You are on placement in a sixth form college. The college has an active LGBTQ society. You are conducting a smoking cessation workshop with the school nurse. The school nurse explains that LGBTQ youth may feel uncomfortable accessing mainstream smoking cessation services and that there is specific guidance available on how best to conduct outreach interviews with LGBTQ communities. During the course of the workshop, the young people tell you they feel targeted by the tobacco industry through social media and the sponsorship of LGBTQ events, suggesting actions are needed that go beyond the individual level to encourage smoking cessation. What would you do to address these practices by tobacco companies?

An outline answer is provided at the end of the chapter.

Chapter summary

In this chapter, we have discussed the specific health needs of diverse communities who often experience worse health, and health outcomes, compared to the general population. Although people are living longer, they are more likely to be living with a preventable disabling condition, which can impact not only on people's quality of life, but has resource implications for nurses and the wider NHS. We have demonstrated how nurses can intervene to improve population health, protect individuals and communities, prevent early mortality, and act on the social determinants that cause inequalities in health.

We have argued that inequalities in health cannot be explained by biology or genetics alone, but also by social determinants (i.e. the conditions in which people are born, live, grow, work and age). The high and variable rates of diseases across non-white ethnic groups (e.g. diabetes and heart disease) are also affected by social determinants, including gender, social class, age, religion and age at migration, suggesting a complex relationship between ethnicity and population health (Nazroo, n.d.). The role of the social determinants is particularly marked in relation to the evidence on inequalities for people with a learning disability.

We have highlighted the transition from communicable diseases (tuberculosis) to non-communicable diseases (Type 2 diabetes) to demonstrate how the changing epidemiology and demography in the UK has given rise to new challenges, including how to deliver health interventions to diverse communities.

The importance of a public health preventative approach in relation to T2D is ever-more pressing given that diabetes is one of the leading causes of lower foot amputation, which can be avoided through appropriate foot care and better management of diabetes. We have demonstrated that in order to avoid the spread of infectious diseases (influenza) and prevent drug resistance to antibiotics (e.g. TB), different models of care or outreach are needed to access those groups most at risk and that are underserved by mainstream services. Collaborative care packages involving agencies in the community are needed to address the social risk factors of TB that can prevent people from prioritising their health, adhering to care plans and completing a course of antibiotics.

An understanding of epidemiology and changing patterns of disease is important to anticipate future trends in order to plan health and social care and associated interventions, which need to be tailored to meet the specific needs of different communities. Tools that allow nurses to profile the local population (see Activity 7.1) in relation to long-term conditions, age, ethnicity and deprivation will be crucial in terms of planning future services and the allocation of resources.

We have discussed the role of evidence-informing policies on tackling inequalities (e.g. the Marmot Review) and provided examples of policies that may exacerbate inequalities (e.g. the spare bedroom subsidy), suggesting that nurses need to be able to exercise political awareness in order to influence policymaking, tackle inequalities and improve nursing care. Nurses who have a better understanding of the health needs of diverse communities will also be able to oppose legislation that discriminates against, and further disadvantages, particular sections of the community by registering their concerns with policy and lawmakers.

Activities: brief outline answers

Activity 7.1   Evidence-based practice and research (pp141–2)

Domain 2: using local authority health profiles to explore areas for health improvement

We chose the London Borough of Tower Hamlets and compared it to another local authority, Eastbourne, to illustrate the differences between the two boroughs and the implications for an intervention. The data were correct as of July 2018.

	Tower Hamlets	**Eastbourne**
Smoking	Levels of smoking in pregnant women at the time of delivery are significantly better than the England average. However, estimated levels of adult smoking are worse than the England average.	Levels of smoking in pregnant women at the time of delivery are worse than the England average. Levels of adult smoking are significantly better than the England average.
Physical activity	The number of physically active adults aged 19+ is not significantly different than the England average.	The number of physically active adults aged 19+ is not significantly different than the England average.
Alcohol-related harm measured in hospital stays	Significantly better than the England average.	Not significantly different than the England average.
Obesity in children	In Year 6, 26.8 per cent of children are classified as obese, worse than the England average.	In Year 6, 17.3 per cent of children are classified as obese, better than the England average.
Diagnosed diabetes	Not significantly different to the England average.	Significantly worse than the England average.
Age 65+	6 per cent.	24.5 per cent.
Ethnicity	53.4 per cent of people come from an ethnic minority group.	2.3 per cent of people come from an ethnic minority group.
Deprivation	One of the 20 per cent most deprived authorities in England, and life expectancy is lower in the most deprived areas.	There are pockets of deprivation. The number of children in low-income families is significantly worse than the England average.
Employment rate	Significantly worse than the England average.	Not significantly different from the England average.
Number of GCSEs	Not significantly different from the England average.	Not significantly different from the England average.

Table 7.4   Tower Hamlets and Eastbourne comparison

Rates of smoking, physical activity and alcohol-related harm in a local authority
compared to the rest of England

At the borough level, adult smoking and childhood obesity would be a priority in Tower
Hamlets. Smoking in pregnancy would be a priority in Eastbourne. However, the data would
need to be considered alongside more local data, including local audits. In 2018, the health profile data on the prevalence of diabetes were not provided. Instead, the data provide a measure of
whether diabetes is diagnosed in primary care by GPs. In this regard, Eastbourne was performing significantly worse than the England average.

How will deprivation, age and ethnic composition influence your choice of a health
improvement intervention?

Different approaches will be needed for different age or ethnic groups. We know that in areas
of deprivation, more outreach approaches may be needed to target specific groups, such as
homeless populations (e.g. see approaches discussed in Activity 7.2). Where deprivation is concentrated in specific areas, approaches that target those areas may be necessary, but targeted
approaches can be problematic as not all poor people live in deprived areas (on proportionate
universalism versus targeted approaches, see Chapter 2).

In areas with black and other minority ethnic groups, as well as ensuring your intervention is culturally and linguistically appropriate, care is needed to ensure it meets diverse populations and is
appropriate to the age, gender, disability and sexual orientation of the people in the community.

Activity 7.2   Critical thinking (p143)

Domain 3: protecting the health of homeless people by improving the uptake of
influenza immunisation

Evidence suggests that people who sleep outside (rough sleepers) are less likely to access primary
healthcare services than the general population and are more likely to attend A&E for healthcare.
Many are not registered with a GP and are not aware of what primary care is offered. Others may fear
discrimination and a negative attitude from staff and other patients attending the practice. An example of how these issues might be addressed through the provision of a dedicated outreach clinic is
provided by the Inclusion Healthcare CIC General Practice Nursing team in Leicester (see **www.eng-
land.nhs.uk/atlas_case_study/practice-nurses-promoting-flu-vaccines-to-the-homeless-community**).

Activity 7.3   Communication (p145)

Domain 4: preventing premature mortality through cancer screening in diverse communities

Guidance for cervical cancer screening for women with a learning disability is available at: **www.
gov.uk/government/publications/cervical-screening-supporting-women-with-learning-disabilities/
supporting-women-with-learning-disabilities-to-access-cervical-screening**

Public Health England has also produced a leaflet to discuss screening with women with learning
disabilities (PHE, 2019). The leaflet is available at: **https://assets.publishing.service.gov.uk/govern
ment/uploads/system/uploads/attachment_data/file/433757/easy-guide-cervical-screening.pdf**

Activity 7.4   Influencing policy (p149)

Influencing policy

You decide to support the LGTBQ youth group to write a letter to their local MP. You can find
out who the local MP is through a website called They Work for You (see the useful websites section at the end of the chapter).

A standard pattern to use when writing a letter to a decision-maker, such as a councillor or MP, is
the EPIC format (see the useful websites section at the end of the chapter). EPIC stands for:

- *Engage*: Say something that is attention-grabbing (e.g. although tobacco advertising has been banned, LGBTQ communities are targeted through social media). These groups are already more likely to smoke compared to other communities. You could write about your own experiences as a nurse working with young people who smoke.
- *Problem*: Explain the precise nature of the problem. How widespread is it? You could ask young people to provide evidence that they are being targeted.
- *Inform*: Inform the MP of what a potential solution to the problem might be (e.g. more resources for smoking cessation activities and stronger legislation).
- *Call to action*: Explain exactly what the MP can do to help. You could ask the MP to write or raise a question in the House of Commons to highlight the problem, which could lead to further policies or legislation banning the targeting of specific communities.

Further reading

Challenge TB (2018) *TB Stigma Measurement Guidance.* Available at: www.challengetb.org/publications/tools/ua/TB_Stigma_Measurement_Guidance.pdf (accessed 20 August 2019).

This report provides guidance on how organisations can carry out TB stigma measurement.

Useful websites

Local Health Authority Profiles

https://fingertips.phe.org.uk/profile/health-profiles

Public Health England's health profile tool.

The Errol McKellar Foundation

http://theerrolmckellarfoundation.com

The Errol McKellar Foundation website.

They Work for You

www.theyworkforyou.com

Use this website to identify your local MP.

How to Write to Your MP

www.results.org.uk/sites/default/files/files/How%20to%20write%20to%20your%20MP_0.pdf

Guidance on how to write to your MP using the EPIC framework.

The National LGB&T Partnership Smoking Cessation Resources

https://nationallgbtpartnership.org/publications/smoking-cessation-resources/

The National LGB&T Partnership's guidelines for local authorities on smoking and LGBT communities.

Pathway: The Faculty

www.pathway.org.uk/faculty/

The Faculty for Homeless and Inclusion Health is an organisation involved in the healthcare of excluded groups, including homeless people, gypsy and traveller communities, sex workers, and vulnerable migrants.

Chapter 8

Mental distress and cultural diversity

Nicky Lambert

NMC Standards of Proficiency for Registered Nurses

This chapter will address the following platforms and proficiencies:

Platform 1: Being an accountable professional

1.14 provide and promote non-discriminatory, person-centred and sensitive care at all times, reflecting on people's values and beliefs, diverse backgrounds, cultural characteristics, language requirements, needs and preferences, taking account of any need for adjustments.

Platform 2: Promoting health and preventing ill health

2.2 demonstrate knowledge of epidemiology, demography, genomics and the wider determinants of health, illness and wellbeing and apply this to an understanding of global patterns of health and wellbeing outcomes.

2.3 understand the factors that may lead to inequalities in health outcomes.

Chapter aims

After reading this chapter, you will be able to:

- explore the factors that impact on the well-being of people with mental health issues who are from minority backgrounds;
- describe ethical practice when working with people with mental health issues; and
- identify your key responsibilities in ensuring best practice when working with people with mental health issues.

Introduction

- In 1914, a psychiatrist at the Georgia State Sanatorium, Dr E.M. Green, published research finding a higher rate of psychosis in African Americans than in their white counterparts; 100 years later, these findings are still resonating in the UK.
- Kirkbride et al. (2008) and Qassem et al. (2015) both identified that people from black and minority ethnic (BME) communities are more likely to experience psychosis than the white majority population, and McManus et al. (2009) found that 3.1 per cent of African Caribbean men have a risk of psychosis, compared 0.2 per cent of white men.
- What is striking about this obvious disparity in the UK is that rates of psychosis in the Caribbean and Africa are not as elevated. This suggests that rather than mental health issues being an inbuilt, genetic hazard for people from BME backgrounds, there are aspects of living as a minority community that put some people at higher risk of mental distress (van Os, 2012).

This chapter begins with the above statistics, which show differences in the well-being of people from BME backgrounds that are both striking and unfair. The issues around mental health and diversity, particularly cultural diversity, are long-standing and emotive. They are also essential for you to understand in order to give compassionate and effective care. This chapter helps you to explore some of the issues around cultural diversity that can affect people's mental health. It also has practical suggestions on working ethically and effectively with all the people in your community.

First, we introduce the idea that language shapes the way that we think, talk and act, and that this in turn has real-world implications for people's health. We then explore the health issues that affect those from minority cultures and their experience of discrimination in health services. We will go on to explore how mental health services can be more accessible and effective in giving care to people from minority backgrounds. The chapter ends with suggestions on how we can give better care as individuals and members of the health service.

The language surrounding diversity can be complicated, but to simplify this discussion we will use Fernando's (2010) definitions of race, culture and ethnicity – words that are often used interchangeably. He describes:

- *race* as characterised by physical appearance (how you look – your skin, hair, features, etc.);
- *culture* as a sociological phenomenon shown in behaviour and attitudes (your actions and beliefs); and
- *ethnicity* as an aspect of identity and a sense of psychological belonging (how you see yourself and who you feel connection to).

It is important to remember that an individual's identity or *sense of self* is often more complex than definitions allow, and that everyone receiving services is an individual who should receive personalised care.

Another idea that you will see in discussions about culture is *minority population*. The social majority are those who dominate positions of power in a society; minority populations are those who do not. A person's minority status might be visible due to religious or cultural dress, or unseen in a condition such as autism. It might be permanent in the form of an individual's ethnicity or temporary such as a mental health issue. A minority population is not defined by numbers, but by proximity and access to social power (e.g. women make up just over half of the UK population but are considered a minority group because of the dominance of men in positions of authority and the social impacts which that entails).

Fernando and Keating (2009) note that people from BME communities are not just more likely to experience mental ill health, but also have worse care. For example, they are more likely to be detained under the Mental Health Act (MHA) and to come into contact with mental health services via the criminal justice system. They note that BME service users are more likely to receive treatment on locked wards and less likely to be referred to counselling and other 'talking therapies'.

There are also variances in this picture between different minority groups. A report by Rehman and Owen (2013) found that while half of the group who were surveyed experienced depression, people with Indian heritage had rates of 61 per cent, while people with African Caribbean backgrounds had rates of between 43 and 44 per cent. A third of the survey participants had experience of anxiety and 16 per cent of respondents reported having schizophrenia. Again, there was disparity, with Caribbean respondents having a rate of 23 per cent and those from Pakistani/Bangladeshi backgrounds reporting lower levels, around 6 per cent.

These findings raise concerns around social justice, prejudice and stigma, as well as diagnosis, treatment and the experience of care in mental health services. It is useful to examine the language commonly used in policy and research to understand and address these issues to provide context to them. You will have encountered the term 'black and minority ethnic' (BME) or 'black, Asian and minority ethnic' (BAME) in health and social documents, so let us explore it.

The term 'BME' describes people belonging to non-white ethnic groups (according to the national census). It is a contested term and is unpopular with some people who find it awkward or officious. In trying to be comprehensive, it covers a range of cultural identities from across Africa, Asia, Europe and the Caribbean by grouping them together as 'non-white'. There are obvious problems suggesting that the only distinguishing or important quality of this range of identities is the shared characteristic of not being defined on a census as white.

The term 'BME' can be used to group someone who is a recent refugee from Sudan with a university student from Dorset who has a grandparent from China. In terms of health and well-being, their needs, concerns and social capital are likely to be very different. While anyone from any minority background may be exposed to stigma, it is probable that someone who is not a native speaker, with limited finances, unfamiliar with cultural norms, and who may have experienced trauma is more likely to be disadvantaged.

Another aspect to this debate is that some documents use 'BAME' in preference to 'BME' as the term specifically recognises the importance of Asian identities within minority communities in Britain. This is a valid point that goes on to highlight all the other marginalised experiences within minority communities. Irish, gypsy, Roma and traveller peoples are sometimes called 'unseen minorities' because while experiencing significant disadvantage in terms of their health, they are not always considered in discussions of BME concerns.

You might wonder why a consideration of language is important to your ability to give compassionate and effective care, but healthcare is embedded in social systems and the health of individuals is shaped directly by the world they experience. Language is key to how we appreciate and address these concerns, and, as a professional working within the Nursing and Midwifery Council code of conduct (NMC, 2015), you have a responsibility to uphold people's dignity, to champion their rights and challenge discrimination. In order to do this, you need to be clear about the factors that can have an impact on the well-being of people with disabilities from minority backgrounds and be able to create supportive health environments.

Understanding the impact of diversity is central to good mental healthcare because an individual's recovery journey can be dependent on active social engagement and a positive sense of self. If someone is excluded because of stigma towards their identity, their return to health is likely to be affected. It is also important to appreciate that culture, heritage, language and religion shape an individual's experience of their own mental health. These factors can also affect the way their friends and family respond to them if they need help, particularly as mental illness can be a source of shame and fear in many cultures (Rehman and Owen, 2013).

Another concern is that despite the changing demographics of BME communities (especially in cities), local health services have sometimes struggled to adapt to provide culturally sensitive care. In order to understand specific needs, to be able to conduct research and to benchmark quality and commission appropriate services, we need ways to describe prevalence, incidence and outcomes for BME communities, so for the moment terminology such as 'BME' remains a practical necessity despite the many issues it raises.

Discrimination in society and within services has been long recognised, and in 2005, the Department of Health's *Delivering Race Equality in Mental Health Care* plan identified 12 characteristics that it was hoped would improve mental healthcare for all by 2010. Areas of action included work to reduce the fear of services in BME communities and to improve service user satisfaction and recovery rates. Another was to reduce the disproportionate numbers of people from BME communities being admitted under the Mental Health Act. There was also a drive to reduce the levels of violence occurring in mental health services. This focused on reducing the practices of restraining and secluding people who became aggressive while mentally distressed, and preventing injury or deaths where restraint proved unavoidable.

Work was also required to improve BME access to talking therapies and to ensure prescriptions of medication were appropriate and effective. The plan also aimed for greater levels of participation by BME communities in co-producing services, policy and professional education. Laws such as the Equality Act 2010 have enabled people to challenge discrimination, and this has moved the dialogue forward around mental distress and diversity; however, there are still very significant injustices experienced by BME communities. Having explored some of these ideas, we will now look at some of the reasons this might be the case in Activity 8.1.

Activity 8.1   Critical thinking

So far, this chapter has established that people from BME communities often have a poorer experience than other sectors of society when it comes to accessing and receiving mental healthcare in the UK. It is a complicated picture, but from your own observations and what you have read, note down some of the reasons that you think might be the cause.

Because these are your own ideas, there is no outline answer provided.

Having looked at your own ideas on why BME communities may have poorer mental health experiences in Activity 8.1, we will now review some of the theories advanced by others. Consider how they agree with your own ideas, as well as where they differ.

Social inequality

BME communities experience higher levels of poverty, increased unemployment and poorer living conditions than the general population (Beasor, 2011; Garrett et al., 2014). These factors are linked to poorer health outcomes (Marmot, 2015) and have proved challenging for health services to address. Public mental health is a growing field, and anti-stigma campaigns such as Time to Change have had some high-profile campaigns, although notably these are less recognised in BME communities (Rehman and Owen, 2013). Like all public health activity, they can be hard to measure in terms of proven outcomes, and are often hindered rather than helped by the political process, short-termism and economic pressures.

Racism and institutionalised racism

Empathy enables us to make the connection between abuse and distress. It seems obvious that facing racism and discrimination could diminish an individual's resilience, as well as that of their community, leading to increased levels of mental distress (Wallace et al., 2016). However, institutionalised racism can prove more challenging to think about. Most people who enter health and social care do so to provide services in a compassionate and respectful way, so it can be hard to appreciate that as a whole, the system can unintentionally produce outcomes that may harm individuals. For example, care pathways designed without stakeholder input, and which are monitored by quality measures that ignore the experience, satisfaction and recovery rates of minority communities, may result in poor outcomes that are overlooked.

People with African Caribbean heritage are up to five times more likely than any other group to be diagnosed and admitted to hospital with psychosis (Mental Health Foundation, 2016). It has been suggested that these higher rates are caused by health professionals making negative assumptions about people, particularly young black men, and pathologising cultural differences. Health provision reflects the society of its time, and there is a disturbing history of problematic power relations within mental healthcare, which includes racism as well as misogyny and homophobia.

Metzl (2010) suggests that black identity became increasingly linked to psychosis as a result of increased social tensions in America as the civil rights protests gained momentum. Indeed, troubling representation of a young black man in an advertisement for an anti-psychotic medication called Haldol from the Archives of General Psychiatry demonstrated at best a fearful and controlling attitude towards black masculinity. This advert, and indeed more about this phenomenon, can be viewed online in articles such as Biaocchi (2011).

Certainly, it is during this time that the diagnostic criteria for schizophrenia in the *Diagnostic and Statistical Manual of Mental Disorders* (which defines and classifies mental illnesses for the American Psychiatric Association) added 'hostility' and 'aggression' as symptoms, a change that, Metzl (2010) states, led to structural racism. As a practice note, do not forget that most countries use the International Statistical Classification of Diseases and Related Health Problems (ICD-10) from the World Health Organization (WHO) for diagnostic criteria, and that there are differences between the two.

We have been exploring the impact of overt racism on mental health; however, stigma can be more subtle in practice. Look at Activity 10.2 and consider how you might respond to it.

Activity 8.2   Critical reflection

The misuse of institutional and professional power has always been with us in society, and one of the most interesting but dangerous aspects of working in mental health is that it sometimes gives you authority to

(Continued)

(Continued)

define what is 'normal' or acceptable and what is not. In order to practise compassionately and ethically, you need to consider how you think about people who are different to you and be reflective about the results of your actions as well as your intentions. How might you handle the following situation?

You hear a colleague saying that a young man from an African background with depression and anxiety isn't suitable for a referral to CBT or talking therapies because he probably couldn't 'think it through as he's more physical'.

Write down your response to this situation.

There are outline answers at the end of the chapter that you may find helpful.

Activity 8.2 is intended to help you to think about ways to manage the power and responsibility that can accompany the privilege of working with people who may be vulnerable due to mental distress. It can be hard sometimes to appreciate the difference between our professional judgement and personal beliefs and prejudices. An example of this occurred when, in 1851, an American, Dr Samuel Cartwright, came across a behaviour that he could not rationally explain and believed that he had discovered a new mental illness. He presented his findings to acclaim in the southern states, suggesting that this 'new' mental illness, drapetomania, was what caused black slaves to run away from captivity (White, 2002).

It seems obvious to us today that an individual attempting to escape slavery is not ill; Cartwright's ideas were met with derision in the North and have never been recognised as part of established diagnoses. I have included them to demonstrate that we can all be blind to our own prejudice and have an obligation to be cautious because our professional judgements can have such serious consequences for other people. Indeed, research by Holland and Ousey (2011) and Weerasinghe (2012) found that even today, just having an accent and wearing dress that signifies a BME identity can make people vulnerable to discrimination.

Another perspective on this issue came from the *Aetiology and Ethnicity in Schizophrenia and Other Psychoses* study – AESOP for short (Morgan et al., 2006). It suggested the hypothesis that experience of urban poverty is what raises the risk of mental distress, not BME identity, and that higher numbers of socially excluded BME communities in urban areas may explain their higher rates of diagnosis. Arguably, this is a rather circular argument, as structural inequalities based on racial discrimination are one of the things confining minority populations to poor housing and limited incomes in the first place.

Fear of mental health services

Most people are treated for mental distress in primary care, and while it is fair to say few people who are referred on to specialist services are enthusiastic about coming into contact with mental health professionals, their trajectory is very different to the 40 per cent of people from BME communities referred through the criminal justice system (Kane, 2014). Certainly, BME communities are over-represented within the criminal justice system, which may account for some of this percentage; however, there are likely to be a number of other factors.

It may be that BME communities are less aware of what help is available (Fernando and Keating, 2009) and struggle to access services if they are not confident English speakers or aware of procedures. Equally, it may well be that they avoid statutory services because of poor previous experiences. It is likely that people avoid services that are not thought to be culturally sensitive or that may bring stigma to individuals and their families (Mereish et al., 2012). It may also be that some communities feel that caregiving is a family responsibility (Cooper et al., 2013), and so they wait until a health issue has become unmanageable in the community (Kane, 2014). Indeed, Morgan et al. (2006) found that not only do some carers from some BME communities delay accessing health services, but when they are forced by necessity to seek statutory help they call the police before a doctor.

The culture of mental health services

We have focused thus far on cultural differences in minority populations, but all groups have beliefs, traditions and attitudes that bind them together. Fernando (2003, 2010) is a key thinker in exploring ideas of cultural dissonance (i.e. the 'culture clash' that can occur between psychiatry and people from non-Western backgrounds).

Psychiatric concepts come from a Western, post-Enlightenment tradition. They are still largely biomedical in focus and contain ideas of 'illness' and 'normality' that may not resonate with BME communities, who may have a more holistic approach or belief in supernatural causations. Health professionals are usually from a background that has had certain privileges, such as access to higher education, status and regular income. This can differentiate them from the people they often end up caring for. There is also an assumption of 'objectivity' in professional identity and the unspoken assumption that diagnosis is a scientific process. This may lead health professionals to over-inflate their confidence in their own judgement rather than encourage them to pause to ask questions and clarify misunderstandings.

Mental health services evolved out of the asylum system, where people who might be a risk to themselves or others were removed from society. The assumed link between 'madness' and danger can result in pressure on professionals to be made responsible for public safety. This can result in professionals who may be risk-averse and who may not always appreciate that sadness, fear and anger can look very different across cultural boundaries.

Cultural differences

There are some cultural practices that specifically impact the well-being of BME communities; they may not be widely sanctioned, but it is good practice to consider them to ensure sensitivity in care provision. Your workplace will have specific policy guidance relating to the safeguarding issues inherent in female genital mutilation (FGM), forced marriage, and what is sometimes called 'honour-based' violence; they are all illegal under UK law. People who have experienced the trauma intrinsic to these issues are likely to have both mental and physical needs, and if you are unsure how best to support a service user in this context, seek advice from your line management.

Politics

One of the most challenging aspects to understanding mental health issues and cultural diversity is what Nutbeam (2004) called 'analysis paralysis'. This occurs where evidence of a problem grows but there is no organised policy implementation to address it. One reason for this is that the current political trajectory in health provision is a neoliberal one. An example of this is that the research linking deprivation to poorer health outcomes – an issue that is key to the well-being of BME communities – has not been translated into meaningful action.

The mental health policy paper *No Health without Mental Health* (Department of Health, 2011) suggests that 'resilience' can protect against mental health difficulties. Larsson (2013) notes that the social impacts of exclusion and deprivation on the health of individuals and their communities are replaced by a vague advice that individuals should be 'mentally tough'. To put this suggestion into perspective, imagine the reaction to a physical health policy that suggested that people at specific risk of ill health could 'will' physical illness away.

Knapp (2012) provides an example of the inadequacy of the mental health commissioning responses to this paper in the rollout of IAPT services (individual psychological interventions). The economic downturn increased social difficulties such as unemployment, and talking therapies, however well delivered, could not offer a practical remedy to these problems. Having counselling services in Job Centres can lead to vulnerable people being held personally responsible for issues caused by broader social problems. For example, in a recession, there are fewer jobs, and people discriminated against because of racism and stigmatised because they have mental health issues may find work harder to obtain. Therapy for these individuals does not change societal ills such as unemployment, but may leave people feeling scapegoated if they struggle to find work.

These factors can seem overwhelming and certainly much bigger than our individual scopes of practice, but understanding them will put you in a position where you can respond to problems in care provision with professional integrity. Your choices not only support the recovery of people in mental distress; they shape the teams you work in. Whether you mean to or not, you act as a role model, and when people see your good practice, that impacts their actions. Policy writing and service commissioning can feel far removed from your everyday work, but policy is written by people – it doesn't just happen! So, it is important that you understand how to make informed decisions and put yourself forward to learn how to participate in this process and shape care for the better. The scenario below is designed to help you consider some of the big ideas we have looked at in a practice context.

Scenario: Working with linguistic diversity

Hibaq Yasin, a 62-year-old woman originally from Somalia, has been feeling dizzy when she stands up suddenly. She talks to her friend who had heart problems after similar symptoms and decides to visit her GP for advice. She hasn't used NHS services since her children were born. She had postnatal depression after the birth of her first child, and she says it was caused by being new in the country, as well as being lonely, with no family near. Her 15-year-old grandson accompanies her as she is very worried about her heart and gets anxious with people she doesn't know. Mrs Yasin can't remember some of the words when she describes her symptoms to the doctor, and her grandson helps her by translating her account of her room spinning when she sat up in bed.

The doctor looks confused, so she demonstrates feeling dizzy and fainting to show him. It is quite dramatic! The GP sees she has a history of mental health issues, so he asks her whether she has any unusual powers or hears voices in her head. Mrs Yasin is baffled but tries to be helpful. When the GP suggests she can see a mental health specialist, she is taken aback and very offended. She says she has never been to a 'mad doctor' and won't go now; she denies having used mental health services when the GP mentions her postnatal depression.

After some confusion, the situation is resolved when Mrs Yasin uses a colloquial expression to describe her dizziness, saying that the room was spinning around her head when she sat up; her grandson mistranslated and told the doctor that her grandmother thought she flew around her bedroom. The doctor asks Mrs Yasin if she thinks she can fly; she giggles and shakes her head. Eventually, Mrs Yasin remembers the word for dizzy and the appointment gets back on track.

The above scenario shows how easy it is for even a straightforward situation such as a consultation for suspected postural hypotension to become complicated when people are talking at cross purposes. Activity 8.3 gives you a chance to respond to the scenario and offer some solutions.

Activity 8.3   Reflection

Critically reflect on the situation described in the above scenario. What factors contributed to the conversation becoming confused?

What could you do to give good care in a situation such as this?

There are some suggested answers at the end of the chapter that you might find helpful.

Activity 8.3 was designed to help you to apply the theories we have explored in the abstract to a practice situation. It was adapted and anonymised from real practice experiences, but unfortunately there have also been real cases that bring together a lot of the ideas we have encountered (NSC NHS Strategic Health Authority, 2003; Prins et al., 1993), as the case study below demonstrates.

Case study: The death of David Bennett

On 30 October 1998, David 'Rocky' Bennett, a 38-year-old African Caribbean man, died after being restrained at a medium secure unit in Norfolk. While the unit had service users from different backgrounds, it was a predominantly culturally white staff group.

Mr Bennett came to the UK when he was 8 years old. He was a Rastafarian who enjoyed drumming; he was offered a traineeship by Chelsea Football Club in his late teens and had worked as a signwriter before being diagnosed with schizophrenia.

At about 10 p.m., an argument between Mr Bennett and another service user arose over the use of the phone. After a struggle, Mr Bennett hit the other service user, who responded with racial abuse. Staff tried to de-escalate the situation but decided to move one of the men overnight to another ward to diffuse the situation. They decided to move Mr Bennett; however, he was aggrieved by this decision as, from his perspective, he had been racially abused and was now being moved as a punishment while the perpetrator was allowed to stay in his room. Mr Bennett became angry when informed that he would be staying overnight and punched a nurse three times, resulting in the restraint by staff that ultimately led to his death.

Mr Bennett was restrained face down on the floor with up to five nurses attempting to hold him. The injuries he sustained during this incident were consistent with excess force. The staff tried to resuscitate him with oxygen, but by the time an ambulance arrived he had been unconscious for 10 minutes. Shortly afterwards, he was pronounced dead.

Findings

- The inquiry into the death of Mr Bennett found no evidence of deliberate misconduct, but the lead nurse was found to be negligent in *not following restraint protocol* to monitor consciousness and manage signs of distress. The restraint was mishandled by the nursing staff, with Mr Bennett's capacity to breathe restricted and the restraint continuing longer than was safe.
- There was *inadequate resuscitation* equipment in the ward, and a doctor, who might have been able to help, took more than an hour to arrive at the clinic.
- There were *irregularities in Mr Bennett's prescription* as he was getting heavy doses of three anti-psychotic drugs. This is poor practice. It was not thought to have been a significant influence on his death; it is, however, likely to have impacted the quality of his life.
- The report noted the *poor treatment of Mr Bennett's family*, who did not receive a timely apology or a timely, transparent account of the incident.
- No evidence of deliberate racism was suggested, and individuals were noted to have been kind. However, the report noted that Mr Bennett's *cultural, social and religious needs had been overlooked* during his time at the clinic.

In 1993, Mr Bennett had written to the nursing director, pointing out:

As you know, there are over half a dozen black boys in this clinic. I don't know if you have realised that there are no Africans on your staff at the moment. We feel there should be at least two black persons in the medical or social work staff. For the obvious reasons of security and contentment for all concerned please do your best to remedy this appalling situation.

(NSC NHS Strategic Health Authority, 2003, p9)

This case was pivotal in mental services changing their approach to cultural diversity, and it led to public debate and service reviews. Staff training and research have improved the management of violence and aggression, and while things are far from perfect, working practices have improved since this report was released. The Promotion of Safe and Therapeutic Services (PSTS) approaches that have been adopted across services and initiatives, such as the Safewards model (Bowers et al., 2015), encourage the use of verbal de-escalation and techniques to support people who are acutely disturbed with greater levels of compassion and safely. Racism and verbal harassment are formally part of risk assessments and seen as triggers for staff to act.

Physical health also continues to grow in importance in mental health settings, and while debates around institutional racism and poor responses to families when things go wrong remain highly charged, these subjects are regular topics for discussion and critique now.

However, it has been over 20 years since Mr Bennett described a lack of diversity in staff, and recent NHS staffing reports confirm this issue as a current concern

(NHS, 2016), with BME staff less likely to be employed or promoted compared to their white counterparts, and more likely to be referred for disciplinary investigation. Research such as *The Snowy White Peaks of the NHS* (Kline, 2014) reiterates these problems and raises the impact that a dearth of BME leadership has on the service as a whole, and on minority communities in particular.

As previously stated, minority communities are varied and their health needs are not static; they can vary in response to life events and across the life span. For example, recent immigrants and asylum seekers are likely to have been exposed to significant uncertainty and anxiety, personal losses, and forced migration. They are at higher risk of having depression, anxiety and post-traumatic stress as a result of being culturally disoriented on reaching the UK, as well being emotionally damaged by experiencing racism and a hostile political system (Latif, 2014). For young, unaccompanied asylum seekers, this situation can be even worse as these stressors are often exacerbated with concerns about their immigration status when they reach adulthood at 18 years.

At the other end of the life course is the experience of BME elders, with Tran et al. (2008) suggesting that older adults from Chinese communities may be underserved as they are less likely to recognise symptoms of mental distress as a health issue, and in systems that require 'self-report' they may be disadvantaged. Johl et al. (2016) found many of these same issues when looking at dementia within BME communities.

Working well with diverse populations is an area that will only grow in importance as at present BME populations are relatively young, but this will change, and the current approach to managing this illness requires early identification and engagement with services. Research on the current prevalence of dementia in UK BME communities is limited, but Truswell (2013) reports that people from African Caribbean backgrounds are more likely to experience vascular dementia, and alongside South Asian and gypsy/traveller communities they have a raised risk of early-onset dementia.

Johl et al.'s (2016) review found that memory loss was commonly viewed as part of ageing rather than as a symptom of mental ill health. They also found that many BME communities saw caring as part of an existing familial responsibility, and Rauf (2011) notes that being an independent carer may be a source of pride for people whose religion may see caring as a God-given 'test'. The carers in this review, who were predominantly female, often had a limited understanding of the support available, and many reported meeting stigma from their communities due to their loved one living with dementia, which impacted on their experiences as carers but also decreased their confidence in accessing services for support.

The intersection of gender and ethnicity may have other impacts on health provision as well; Latif (2014) states that women from minority communities may present with somatic or physical symptoms of mental distress rather than emotional or psychological ones. This could be because of concerns about being stigmatised; it could be that they conceptualise their experiences differently or just have little experience of Western biomedical models of health.

The issues that we have considered in this chapter have all been big and complex – racism, identity, culture and stigma – and trying to address them can feel overwhelming; however, there are lots of things that you can do to make the support that you give better.

Activity 8.4   Decision-making

When you work with people across a range of backgrounds, consider your own practice. What decisions do you make that help people from diverse communities experience good care? Have a look the list in the next section and think about skills you already have, and consider ways to improve your practice. Remember to note the things you do well already, as well as the things you may need to read up on or do differently.

As this answer is based on your own observation, there is no outline answer at the end of the chapter.

Best practice for working with people from minority communities in mental distress

As an individual practitioner, considering the following will help you to practise confidently when working with people from minority communities in mental distress.

Your attitude

Providing care for people is a privilege, and to do that well you will need to know about the lives and experiences of people who are different from you. Push yourself to engage with films, books and art that help you to see things from other people's perspectives.

Being culturally competent involves you being open-minded and working to inform yourself about the lives of those you are supporting. You should consider a person's background as well as their individuality to avoid pathologising personal and cultural preferences.

Your knowledge

Make sure that you are aware of the ways that people from culturally diverse backgrounds might talk about or show mental distress. If a service user is described to you as paranoid, for example, consider that behaviour in light of social realities, and be someone that people are able to talk to about any form of stigma that they might experience.

Be prepared to tolerate some uncertainty when trying to understand other people's experiences and learn to cultivate humility with regard to the limits of your personal and professional understanding. Ask for help when you need it!

Be aware of the rights of service users and address any stigma or discrimination you are aware of. This might mean supporting an individual to complain, contacting an advocate, or speaking up on behalf of someone. Anyone can raise a concern if they feel the safety of patients or the public is at risk (NMC, 2019). Your workplace will also have a policy, and you should contact your union if you have concerns as to how your speaking up may be received.

Professional approaches

Personalisation means that we adapt to the needs of the individual rather than assuming 'one size fits all'. It is a way of working with a *strengths-based model,* where care builds on people's autonomy, resilience and abilities rather than making assumptions about what is best for someone from beliefs based on their diagnosis.

Care is given in a social context and it is important that professionals provide *holistic care.* This means making sure that you look beyond the bio-medical model and factor in the impact of disadvantage and unmet needs on someone's experience when you are caring for them.

As a service, we should be considering the following in order to better support people from minority communities in mental distress.

Co-production

Co-production moves care provision on from tokenistic service user involvement to bringing stakeholder expertise into the core of decision-making and agenda-setting of the service. This can include anything from supporting service users to evaluate the services they use, to capacity-building by including peer mentors as part of the workforce. Statutory services can also help provide the infrastructure to develop *communities of interest.* They are well placed to forge links with a range of specialist and community-based organisations. Many voluntary organisations provide flexible and tailored services that support the mental and physical health of BME communities; however, funding is rarely secure for long, which can undermine their efforts. A *community of interest* between statutory and voluntary partners can share intelligence, work together to provide an evidence base for best practice, work as advocates, and act as a reference point.

Commissioning and research

We can work with service users and researchers to commission an *evidence base* for best practice in supporting the mental health of BME communities. Commissioning agreements should be formulated to ensure that services collect routine data on outcomes for BME communities so that we can benchmark services to identify good practice to share (Mind, 2013).

Given the historically poor relationship between mental health services and BME communities, *public mental health initiatives* could be designed to reach this community, tackling stigma around mental distress and signposting people towards help. The inequalities that exist around BME populations and mental healthcare cannot be explained by a 'variable disease burden' model, and we need a better understanding of the experience and outcomes of mental health treatment among BME groups. We would benefit from a clear research and action plan. Indeed, in light of the harm caused by stigma and discrimination more generally, there is also a case to suggest that racism itself should be treated as a public health issue because of the impact it has on people's well-being, and action taken to address it.

Chapter summary

- In this chapter, we have looked at some of the terminology associated with mental distress and cultural diversity and explored its context.
- We have considered the factors that impact on the well-being of people with mental health issues who are from minority backgrounds.
- Activities have shown how theories can be used to inform ethical practice, and we have explored how you can ensure best practice when working with people from minority communities with mental health issues.

Activities: brief outline answers

Activity 8.2   Critical reflection (pp159–60)

First, it is more respectful of others' clinical opinion not to rush to judgement as they might be absolutely correct but just expressing themselves poorly. However, you could probe and ask why they think that, and note that a talking therapy would normally be recommended here. A short conversation should let you know where things stand.

If you think that a service user is being denied services based on discrimination, you need to report it. It may be that you have the kind of relationship with your colleague where you can talk to them about things privately and raise your concern. If that is not the case, you will need to speak to your line manager; if you are not satisfied with the response, follow your reporting procedure and seek support from your union if need be.

The best solution would be a strong service user advocacy presence in your service from the start and clear pathways that are transparent and available to all, so that service users are aware of their options and can more fully participate in their care. When we write our notes, hand over to colleagues or express professional opinions, we need to be clear that our goal is only to support that individual to recover – our prejudices are not helpful in doing that, and our first duty is always to the people we serve.

Activity 8.3   Reflection (p164)

What factors contributed to the conversation becoming confused?

You may have answers that are not listed below; it's not an exhaustive list, but there seem to have been a number of misconceptions and misunderstandings.

The first is around translation; getting people who can translate in practice can be tricky, but there are telephone and online services that can help. There are also gender and age dynamics to consider; at 15 years, Hibaq's grandson is still legally a child. He is also male, and both of these factors may affect what Hibaq is comfortable saying in front of him. You should consider managing any pressure on him in this interaction. It is also a mistake to assume that people speak the same language and specific dialects as their family members.

The second point is about beliefs around illness. Mrs Yasin has come to the appointment anxious and fearful; these emotions should be addressed as they can impact on communication. She has described her symptomology using strong imagery and by demonstrating physically – unfortunately, these visuals have provoked surprise rather than understanding! There are expectations of formal interactions that differ between people; we only usually consider them when one party steps outside them. Mrs Yasin has been well for many years, and while there is no reason to assume postnatal depression would be followed up 40 years later by psychosis, it is interesting that a past history of mental distress can colour any new assessment. It is also notable that Mrs Yasin did not see her postnatal depression as a mental health issue, but a social one to do with being newly arrived in a new situation and isolated from former systems of support. As she received her care while in maternity services, it is likely that she thinks she hasn't had contact with mental health workers.

What could you do to give good care in a situation such as this?

Ensure that you follow best practice guidance when using an interpreter and be mindful of the things that can go wrong.

Be respectful and friendly – therapeutic communication can be complicated and run into problems, but developing warmth and trust in your interactions will only help.

Be aware of body language and verbal cues – if you sense that someone doesn't understand you, stop and clarify. People may use different ways of displaying fear, sadness and anger, and in some cases physical expression of this kind is frowned upon, so always check!

Further reading

Haith, M. (2017) *Understanding Mental Health Practice.* London: Learning Matters.

This book outlines the fundamentals of mental healthcare, equipping you with essential knowledge around what is meant by mental health and well-being, common mental health problems, and typical interventions and treatment options.

Kline, R. (2015) *Beyond the Snowy White Peaks of the NHS? Diversity in the NHS.* Available at: https://raceequalityfoundation.org.uk/wp-content/uploads/2018/02/Health-Briefing-39-_Final.pdf (accessed 20 August 2019).

This report provides an overview of diversity within health staff and its impact on care.

Race Equality Foundation (2015) *Better Practice in Mental Health for Black and Minority Ethnic Communities.* Available at: http://raceequalityfoundation.org.uk/wp-content/uploads/2018/10/Better-practice-in-mental-health.pdf (accessed 20 August 2019).

This report explores the research base and policy content around the mental health of BME communities, and highlights lessons that can be learned from voluntary and community sector organisations working with these communities.

Useful websites

Race Equality Foundation

https://raceequalityfoundation.org.uk

Exploring discrimination and disadvantage, and using that knowledge to help overcome barriers and promote race equality in health, housing and social care.

References

Abbott, C., Chaturvedi, N., Malik, R., Salgami, E., Yates, A., Pemberton, P., et al. (2010) Explanations for the lower rates of diabetic neuropathy in Indian Asians versus Europeans. *Diabetes Care*, 33(6): 1325–30.

Acheson, D. (1988) *Public Health in England: The Report of the Committee of Inquiry into the Future Development of the Public Health Function.* London: HMSO.

Adekoya, A.A. and Ogunola, A.A. (2015) Relationship between left-handedness and increased intelligence among university intelligence among university graduates. *Psychology and Behavioural Sciences*, 4(2): 44–50.

Ali, M. (2017) Communication skills 1: benefits of effective communication for patients. *Nursing Times*, 113(12): 18–19.

Ali, M. (2018) Communication skills 3: non-verbal communication. *Nursing Times*, 114(2): 41–2.

Alslman, E.T., Ahmad, M.M., Bani Hani, M.A. and Atiyeh, H.M. (2015) Health: a developing concept in nursing. *International Journal of Nursing Knowledge*, 28(2): 64–9.

Andrews, N., Greenfield, S., Drever, W. and Redwood, S. (2017) Strong, female and black: stereotypes of African Caribbean women's body shape and their effects on clinical encounters. *Health*, 21(2): 189–204.

Anonymous (2016) *Communication in the Real World: An Introduction to Communication Studies.* Available at: http://open.lib.umn.edu/communication/ (accessed 28 April 2018).

Aquino, M.R.J.V., Edge, D. and Smith, D.M. (2015) Pregnancy as an ideal time for intervention to address the complex needs of black and minority ethnic women: views of British midwives. *Midwifery*, 31(3): 373–9.

Argyle, M., Salter, V., Nicholson, H., Williams, M. and Burgess, P. (1970) The communication of inferior and superior attitudes by verbal and non-verbal signals. *British Journal of Social and Clinical Psychology*, 9: 221–31.

Ashley, W. (2014) The angry black woman: the impact of pejorative stereotypes on psychotherapy with black women. *Social Work in Public Health*, 29: 27–34.

Ashworth, A. (n.d.) *Sexual Orientation: A Guide for the NHS.* Available at: www.stonewall.org.uk/sites/default/files/stonewall-guide-for-the-nhs-web.pdf (accessed 20 August 2019).

Aspinall, P.J. (2014) *Hidden Needs Identifying Key Vulnerable Groups in Data Collections: Vulnerable Migrants, Gypsies and Travellers, Homeless People, and Sex Workers.* Available at: https://assets.

publishing.service.gov.uk/government/uploads/system/uploads/attachment_data/ file/287805/vulnerable_groups_data_collections.pdf (accessed 16 August 2018).

Bach, S. and Grant, A. (2015) *Communication and Interpersonal Skills in Nursing* (3rd edn). London: SAGE.

Bachmann, C.L. and Gooch, R. (2019) *LGBT in Britain: Health Report*. Available at: www. stonewall.org.uk/lgbt-britain-health (accessed 6 October 2019).

Baggott, R. (2011) *Public Health Policy and Politics*. London: Palgrave Macmillan.

Baillie, L. (2017) An exploration of the 6Cs as a set of values for nursing practice. *British Journal of Nursing*, 26(10): 558–63.

Baillie, L. and Matiti, M. (2013) Dignity, equality and diversity: an exploration of how discriminatory behaviour of healthcare workers affects patient dignity. *Diversity & Equality in Health & Care*, 10(1): 5–12.

Baker, M. (2016) Detecting pressure damage in people with darkly pigmented skin. *Wound Essentials*, 11(1): 28–31.

Ballantyne, H. (2016) Developing nursing care plans. *Nursing Standard*, 30(26): 51–7.

Barrett, D., Wilson, B. and Woollands, A. (2019) *Care Planning: A Guide for Nurses* (3rd edn). London: Routledge.

Bauld, L. (2011) *The Impact of Smoking Free Legislation in England: Evidence Review*. Available at: https://assets.publishing.service.gov.uk/government/uploads/system/ uploads/attachment_data/file/216319/dh_124959.pdf (accessed 3 September 2019).

BBC News (2018) *Restrictions Lifted on Dartford Nurse Who Gave Bible to Patient*. Available at: www.bbc.co.uk/news/uk-england-kent-45115124 (accessed 1 June 2019).

Beasor, S. (2011) *Housing Benefit and Welfare Reform: Impact of the Proposed Changes on Black and Minority Ethnic Communities*. Available at: www.hqnetwork.org.uk/scripts/get_ normal?file=7290 (accessed 2 May 2017).

Bell, R. (2017) *Psychosocial Pathways and Health Outcomes: Informing Action on Health Inequalities*. London: PHE.

Benbow, W. and Jordan, G. (2016) *A Handbook for Student Nurses: Introducing Key Issues Relevant for Practice*. Banbury: Lantern.

Berlin, E.A. and Fowkes, W.C. (1983) A teaching framework for cross-cultural health care: application in family practice. *Western Journal of Medicine*, 39(6): 934–8.

Bettancourt, J.R., Green, A.R., Carrillo, J.E. and Ananeh-Firempong, O. (2003) Defining cultural competence: a practical framework for addressing racial/ethnic disparities in health and health care. *Public Health Reports*, 118: 293–302.

Bhopal, K. (2018) *White Privilege: The Myth of a Post-Racial Society*. Bristol: Policy Press.

Biaocchi, A. (2011) The racialization of mental illness. *Jezebel*. Available at: https://jezebel. com/the-racialization-of-mental-illness-5804717 (accessed 24 October 2019).

Bjarnason, D., Mick, J., Thompson, J.A. and Cloyd, E. (2009) Perspectives on transcultural care. *Nursing Clinics*, 44(4): 495–503.

Blom, N., Huijts, T. and Kraaykamp, G. (2016) Ethnic health inequalities in Europe: the moderating and amplifying role of healthcare system characteristics. *Social Science & Medicine*, 158: 43–51.

Bloomfield, J. and Pegram, A. (2015) Care, compassion and communication. *Nursing Standard*, 29(25): 45–50.

Booker, C.L., Rieger, G. and Unger, J.B. (2017) Sexual orientation health inequality: evidence from *Understanding Society*, the UK longitudinal household study. *Preventive Medicine*, 101: 126–32.

Bowers, L., James, K., Quirk, A., Simpson, A., Stewart, D. and Hodsoll, J. (2015) Reducing conflict and containment rates on acute psychiatric wards: the Safewards cluster randomised controlled trial. *International Journal of Nursing Studies*, 52(9): 1412–22.

Bradby, H. and Brand, T. (2016) *Dimensions of Diversity: Terminology in Health Research.* IRiS Working Paper Series, No. 12/2015 (UPWEB Working Paper Series, No. 1/2016). Birmingham: Institute for Research into Superdiversity.

Braedel-Kühner, C. and Müller, A. (2015) *Re-Thinking Diversity: Multiple Approaches in Theory, Media, Communities, and Managerial Practice.* New York: Springer.

Briggs, A., Mytton, O., Kehlbacher, A., Tiffin, R., Elhussein, A. and Rayner, M. (2013) Health impact assessment of the UK Soft Drinks Industry Levy: a comparative risk assessment modelling study. *The Lancet*, 2(1): E15–22.

Bristowe, K., Hodson, M., Wee, B., Almack, K., Johnson, K., Daveson, B.A., et al. (2018) Recommendations to reduce inequalities for LGBT people facing advanced illness: ACCESSCare national qualitative interview study. *Palliative Medicine*, 32(1): 23–35.

Bucknor-Ferron, P. and Zagaja, L. (2016) Five strategies to combat unconscious bias. *Nursing*, 46(11): 61–2.

Burchardt, T., Obolenskaya, P., Vizard, P. and Battaglini, M. (2018) *Experience of Multiple Disadvantage among Roma, Gypsy and Traveller Children in England and Wales.* London: LSE.

Burford, B., Worrow, E. and Caspary, A. (2009) *Religion or Belief: A Practical Guide for the NHS.* London: Department of Health.

Burnard, P. (1992) *Know Yourself! Self-Awareness Activities for Nurses.* London: Scutari.

Burnard, P. and Gill, P. (2014) *Culture, Communication and Nursing.* London: Routledge.

Burnes, D.P., Antle, B.J., Williams, C.C. and Cook, L. (2008) Mothers raising children with sickle cell disease at the intersection of race, gender, and illness stigma. *Health & Social Work*, 33(3): 211–20.

Burnham, J., Palmer, D.A. and Whitehouse, L. (2008) Learning as a context for differences and differences as a context for learning. *Journal of Family Therapy and Systemic Practice*, 30: 529–42.

Burrell, R.R. (2019) *The Black Majority Church: Exploring the Impact of Faith and a Faith Community on Mental Health and Well-Being.* Doctoral dissertation, Middlesex University/ Metanoia Institute.

Campinha-Bacote, J. (2002) The process of cultural competence in the delivery of health-care services: a model of care. *Journal of Transcultural Nursing*, 13(3): 181–4.

Campinha-Bacote, J. (2011) *Delivering Patient-Centred Care in the Midst of a Cultural Conflict: The Role of Cultural Competence*. Available at: http://ojin.nursingworld.org/ MainMenuCategories/ANAMarketplace/ANAPeriodicals/OJIN/TableofContents/Vol-16-2011/No2-May-2011/Delivering-Patient-Centered-Care-in-the-Midst-of-a-Cultural-Conflict.html (accessed 13 August 2018).

Cancer Research UK (2018) *Breast Cancer Incidence (Invasive)*. Available at: www.cancer-researchuk.org/health-professional/cancer-statistics/statistics-by-cancer-type/breast-cancer#heading-Zero (accessed 19 August 2018).

Candler, T., Mahmoud, O., Lynn, R., Majbar, A., Barrett, T. and Shield, J. (2018) Continuing risk of Type 2 diabetes incidence in children and young people in the UK. *Diabetic Medicine*, 35: 737–44.

Caraher, M. and Perry, I. (2017) Sugar, salt, and the limits of self-regulation in the food industry. *BMJ*, 357: j1709.

Caraher, M., Lloyd, S. and Madelin, T. (2014) The 'school foodshed': schools and fast-food outlets in a London borough. *British Food Journal*, 116(3): 472–93.

Catalano, J.T. (2015) *Nursing Now! Today's Issues, Tomorrow's Trends*. Philadelphia, PA: FA Davis.

Celeste, L., Meeussen, L., Verschueren, K. and Phalet, K. (2016) Minority acculturation and peer rejection: costs of acculturation misfit with peer-group norms. *British Journal of Social Psychology*, 55(3): 544–63.

Centers for Disease Control and Prevention (2011) *National Diabetes Fact Sheet, 2011*. Available at: www.cdc.gov/diabetes/pubs/pdf/ndfs_2011.pdf (accessed 3 September 2019).

Centers for Disease Control and Prevention (2014) *NCHHSTP Social Determinants of Health*. Available at: www.cdc.gov/nchhstp/socialdeterminants/definitions.html (accessed 29 August 2019).

Chaffee, M.W., Mason, D.J. and Leavitt, J.K. (2012) A framework for action in policy and politics. In D.J. Mason, J.K. Leavitt and M.W. Chaffee (eds), *Policy and Politics in Nursing and Healthcare* (6th edn). St Louis, MO: Elsevier Saunders.

Challenge TB (2018) *TB Stigma Measurement Guidance*. Available at: www.challengetb.org/ publications/tools/ua/TB_Stigma_Measurement_Guidance.pdf (accessed 20 August 2019).

Chambers, S. (2003) Use of non-verbal communication skills to improve nursing care. *British Journal of Nursing*, 12(14): 874–8.

Cheraghi, M.A., Manookian, A. and Nasrabadi, A.N. (2014) Human dignity in religion-embedded cross-cultural nursing. *Nursing Ethics*, 21(8): 916–28.

Chesney, E. Goodwin, G.M. and Fazel, S. (2014) Risks of all-cause and suicide mortality in mental disorders: a meta-review. *World Psychiatry*, 13: 153–60.

Chopra, D. (2012) *Spiritual Solutions: Answers to Life's Greatest Challenges*. New York: Harmony.

Christiansen, A., O'Brien, M.R., Kirton, J.A., Zubairu, K. and Bray, L. (2015) Delivering compassionate care: the enablers and barriers. *British Journal of Nursing*, 24(16): 833–7.

Clark, F. (2014) Discrimination against LGBT people triggers health concerns. *The Lancet*, 383(9916): 500–2.

Clarke, J. (2016) Spiritual care. In D. Sellman and P. Snelling (eds), *Becoming a Nurse: Fundamentals of Professional Practice for Nursing*. London: Routledge.

Clarridge, A. (2017) Spirituality: a neglected aspect of care. In S. Chilton, H. Bain, A. Clarridge and K. Melling (eds), *A Textbook of Community Nursing* (2nd edn). London: Routledge.

Codjoe, L., Barber, S. and Thornicroft, G. (2019) Tackling inequalities: a partnership between mental health services and black faith communities. *Journal of Mental Health*, 28(3): 225–8.

Collins, P.H. and Bilge, S. (2016) *Intersectionality*. Hoboken, NJ: John Wiley & Sons.

Cooper, J., Steeg, S., Webb, R., Stewart, S.L., Applegate, E., Hawton, K., et al. (2013) Risk factors associated with repetition of self-harm in black and minority ethnic (BME) groups: a multi-centre cohort study. *Journal of Affective Disorders*, 148(2): 435–9.

Coulter, A. (2011) *Engaging Patients with Healthcare*. Berkshire: Open University Press.

Craig, G.M., Booth, H., Hall, J., Story, A., Hayward, A., Goodburn, A., et al. (2008) Establishing a new service role in tuberculosis care: the tuberculosis link worker. *Journal of Advanced Nursing*, 61(4): 413–24.

Crawford, T., Candlin, S. and Roger, P. (2015) *New Perspectives on Understanding Cultural Diversity in Nurse–Patient Communication*. Available at: www.collegianjournal.com/article/S1322-7696(15)00078-5/pdf (accessed 1 November 2018).

Crenshaw, K. (1989) Demarginalizing the intersection of race and sex: a black feminist critique of antidiscrimination doctrine, feminist theory and antiracist politics. *University of Chicago Legal Forum*, 1(8): 139–67.

Cromarty, H. (2018) *Gypsies and Travellers*. Briefing Paper, House of Commons Library, Number 08083, 8 May 2018. Available at: https://researchbriefings.parliament.uk/ResearchBriefing/Summary/CBP-8083 (accessed 29 September 2019).

Culley, L. (2010) Exclusion and inclusion: unequal lives and unequal health. *Journal of Research in Nursing*, 15(4): 299–301.

Darzi, Lord (2008) *Department of Health: High Quality Care for All – NHS Next Stage Review Final Report*. Available at: https://assets.publishing.service.gov.uk/government/uploads/system/uploads/attachment_data/file/228836/7432.pdf (accessed 21 October 2019).

Dein, S. (2006) Race, culture and ethnicity in minority research: a critical discussion. *Journal of Cultural Diversity*, 13(2), 68–75.

Dein, S., Cook, C.C.H. and Koenig, H. (2012) Religion, spirituality, and mental health: current controversies and future directions. *Journal of Nervous and Mental Disease*, 200(10): 852–5.

Department for Business, Innovation and Skills (2012) *Skills for Life Survey: A Survey of Literacy, Numeracy and ITC Levels in England*. Available at: https://assets.publishing.service.

gov.uk/government/uploads/system/uploads/attachment_data/file/36000/12-p168-2011-skills-for-life-survey.pdf (accessed 28 April 2018).

Department for Communities and Local Government (DCLG) (2012) *Progress Report by the Ministerial Working Group on Tackling Inequalities Experienced by Gypsies and Travellers.* Available at: https://assets.publishing.service.gov.uk/government/uploads/system/uploads/attachment_data/file/6287/2124046.pdf (accessed 25 October 2019).

Department of Health (2001) *Valuing People: A New Strategy for Learning Disability for the 21st Century.* Available at: https://assets.publishing.service.gov.uk/government/uploads/system/uploads/attachment_data/file/250877/5086.pdf (accessed 28 April 2018).

Department of Health (2005) *Delivering Race Equality in Mental Health Care: An Action Plan For Reform Inside and Outside Services and the Government's Response to the Independent Inquiry into the Death of David Bennett.* Available at: http://webarchive. nationalarchives.gov.uk/20130107105354/http:/www.dh.gov.uk/en/publications andstatistics/publications/publicationspolicyandguidance/dh_4100773 (accessed 2 May 2017).

Department of Health (2009) *Religion or Belief: A Practical Guide for the NHS.* Available at: https://webarchive.nationalarchives.gov.uk/20130123195548/http://www.dh.gov. uk/en/Publicationsandstatistics/Publications/PublicationsPolicyAndGuidance/ DH_093133 (accessed 30 January 2019).

Department of Health (2010a) *Essence of Care: Benchmarks for Communication.* London: Available at: https://assets.publishing.service.gov.uk/government/uploads/system/ uploads/attachment_data/file/216695/dh_119973.pdf (accessed 9 December 2019).

Department of Health (2010b) *Our Health and Wellbeing Today.* Available at: https:// assets.publishing.service.gov.uk/government/uploads/system/uploads/attachment_ data/file/215911/dh_122238.pdf (accessed 6 October 2019).

Department of Health (2011) *No Health without Mental Health: A Cross-Government Mental Health Outcomes Strategy for People of All Ages.* Available at: www.gov.uk/government/uploads/ system/uploads/attachment_data/file/213761/dh_124058.pdf (accessed 2 May 2017).

Department of Health (2012a) *Compassion in Practice: Nursing, Midwifery and Care Staff – Our Vision and Strategy.* Available at: www.england.nhs.uk/wp-content/uploads/2012/12/ compassion-in-practice.pdf (accessed 6 October 2019).

Department of Health (2012b) *The New Public Health Role of Local Authorities.* Available at: https://assets.publishing.service.gov.uk/government/uploads/system/uploads/ attachment_data/file/213009/Public-health-role-of-local-authorities-factsheet.pdf (accessed 3 September 2019).

Department of Health (2013) *Report of the Mid Staffordshire NHS Foundation Trust Public Enquiry Volume 3: Present and Future.* Available at: https://assets.publishing.service.gov. uk/government/uploads/system/uploads/attachment_data/file/279121/0898_iii.pdf (accessed 13 September 2018).

Department of Health (2015a) *NHS Constitution.* Available at: www.gov.uk/government/ publications/the-nhs-constitution-for-england/the-nhs-constitution-for-england (accessed 1 July 2018).

Department of Health (2015b) *Prime Minister's Challenge on Dementia 2020.* Available at: www.gov.uk/government/publications/prime-ministers-challenge-on-dementia-2020/ prime-ministers-challenge-on-dementia-2020 (accessed 3 September 2019).

DeWilde, C. and Burton, W. (2017) Cultural distress: an emerging paradigm. *Journal of Transcultural Nursing,* 28(4): 334–41.

Douglas, M.K., Rosenkoetter, M., Pacquiao, D.F., Callister, L.C., Hattar-Pollara, M., Lauderdale, J., et al. (2014) Guidelines for implementing culturally competent nursing care. *Journal of Transcultural Nursing,* 25(2): 109–21.

Dovidio, J.F. and Fiske, S.T. (2012) Under the radar: how unexamined biases in decision-making processes in clinical interactions can contribute to health care disparities. *American Journal of Public Health,* 102(5): 945–52.

Dovidio, J.F., Esses, V.M., Glick, P. and Hewstone, M. (2010) *The SAGE Handbook of Prejudice, Stereotyping and Discrimination.* London: SAGE.

DR Barometer (n.d.) *The Diabetic Retinopathy Barometer Report: Global Findings.* Available at: www.iapb.org/wp-content/uploads/DR-Global-Report-1.pdf (accessed 21 October 2019).

Drewniak, D., Krones, T. and Wild, V. (2017) Do attitudes and behaviour of health care professionals exacerbate health care disparities among immigrant and ethnic minority groups? An integrative literature review. *International Journal of Nursing Studies,* 70: 89–98.

Duncan, P. (2017) Gay relationships are still criminalised in 72 countries, report finds. *The Guardian,* 27 July 2017. Available at: www.theguardian.com/world/2017/jul/27/gay-relationships-still-criminalised-countries-report (accessed 16 August 2018).

Dyer, C. (2018) *NHS Failed to Communicate Feeding Advice to Refugee Mother, Court Rules.* Available at: www.bmj.com/content/361/bmj.k1711 (accessed 28 April 2018).

Emerson, E. and Baines, S. (2011) Health inequalities and people with learning disabilities in the UK. *Tizard Learning Disability Review,* 16(1): 42–8.

Emerson, E., Glover, G., Turner, S., Greig, R., Hatton, C., Baines, S., et al. (2012) Improving health and lives: the learning disabilities public health observatory. *Advances in Mental Health and Intellectual Disabilities,* 6(1): 26–32.

Emerson, E., Robertson, J., Baines, S. and Hatton, C. (2014) The self-rated health of British adults with intellectual disability. *Research in Developmental Disabilities,* 35(3): 591–6.

Emerson, E., Hatton, C., Baines, S. and Robertson, J. (2016) The physical health of British adults with intellectual disability: cross sectional study. *International Journal for Equity in Health,* 15(1): 11.

Equality Act (2010) *Equality Act 2010: Guidance.* Available at: www.gov.uk/guidance/ equality-act-2010-guidance (accessed 5 September 2019).

Equality and Human Rights Commission (EHRC) (2016a) *England's Most Disadvantaged Groups: Gypsies, Travellers and Roma.* Available at: www.equalityhumanrights.com/sites/ default/files/is-england-fairer-2016-most-disadvantaged-groups-gypsies-travellers-roma. pdf (accessed 25 October 2019).

Equality and Human Rights Commission (EHRC) (2016b) *Healing a Divided Britain: The Need for a Comprehensive Race Strategy.* Available at: https://www.equalityhumanrights.com/

en/publication-download/healing-divided-britain-need-comprehensive-race-equality-strategy (accessed 9 December 2019).

Equality and Human Rights Commission (EHRC) (2017) *Gypsies and Travellers: Simple Solutions for Living Together*. Available at: www.equalityhumanrights.com/en/gypsies-and-travellers-simple-solutions-living-together (accessed 14 August 2018).

Everett, J.S., Budescu, M. and Sommers, M.S. (2012) Making sense of skin color in clinical care. *Clinical Nursing Research*, 21(4): 495–516.

Fenton, K. (2016) *Working Globally to Tackle Non-Communicable Diseases*. Available at: https://publichealthmatters.blog.gov.uk/2016/02/09/working-globally-to-tackle-non-communicable-diseases/ (accessed 3 April 2019).

Fernando, S. (2003) *Cultural Diversity, Mental Health and Psychiatry: The Struggle against Racism*. Hove: Brunner-Routledge.

Fernando, S. (2010) *Mental Health: Race and Culture* (3rd edn). London: Palgrave Macmillan.

Fernando, S. and Keating, F. (eds) (2009) *Mental Health in a Multi-Ethnic Society: A Multidisciplinary Handbook* (2nd edn). London: Routledge.

Fish, J. and Evans, D. (2016) Promoting cultural competency in nursing care of LGBT patients. *Journal of Research in Nursing*, 21(3): 159–62.

Fitchett, G. (2017) Recent progress in chaplaincy-related research. *Journal of Pastoral Care & Counseling*, 71(3): 163–75.

FitzGerald, C. and Hurst, S. (2017) Implicit bias in healthcare professionals: a systematic review. *BMC Medical Ethics*, 18(1): 19.

Flowers, D. (2014) *Culturally Competent Nursing Care: A Challenge for the 21st Century*. Available at: http://citeseerx.ist.psu.edu/viewdoc/download?doi=10.1.1.571.300&rep=rep1&type=pdf (accessed 2 September 2019).

Foundation for People with Learning Disabilities (2019) *Learning Disability Statistics: Mental Health Problems*. Available at: www.mentalhealth.org.uk/learning-disabilities/help-information/learning-disability-statistics-/187699 (accessed 30 June 2019).

Fredrickson, G.M. (2015) Models of American ethnic relations: a historical perspective. In *Diverse Nations: Explorations in the History of Racial and Ethnic Pluralism*. London: Routledge.

Friedlander, D., Trinh, Q.-D., Krasnova, A., Lipsitz., S., Sun, M., Nguyen, P., et al. (2018) Racial disparity in delivering definitive therapy for intermediate/high-risk localised prostate cancer: the impact of facility features and socioeconomic characteristics. *European Urology*, 73: 445–51.

Frost, D.M. (2011) Social stigma and its consequences for the socially stigmatized. *Social and Personality Psychology Compass*, 5(11): 824–39.

Fukada, M. (2018) Nursing competency: definition, structure and development. *Yonago Acta Medica*, 61: 1–7.

Gandy, M. (2003) Life without germs: contested episodes in the history of tuberculosis. In M. Gandy and A. Zumla (eds), *The Return of the White Plague*. London: Verso.

Garner, S. (2017) *Racism: An Introduction* (2nd edn). London: SAGE.

Garrett, H. Piddington, J. and Nicol, S. (2014) *The Housing Conditions of Minority Ethnic Households in England.* Available at: www.better-housing.org.uk/briefings/ housingconditionsminorityethnic-households-england (accessed 2 May 2017).

General Medical Council (GMC) (2019) *Ethical Guidance: Treatment and Care Towards the End of Life: Good Practice in Decision-Making.* Available at: www.gmc-uk.org/ethical-guidance/ethical-guidance-for-doctors/treatment-and-care-towards-the-end-of-life/ guidance (accessed 13 October 2019).

Giddens, A. and Sutton, P.W. (2017) *Sociology* (8th edn). Cambridge: Polity Press.

Giger, J. and Davidhizar, R. (2002) The Giger and Davidhizar transcultural assessment model. *Journal of Transcultural Nursing,* 13: 185–8.

Gilbert, L., Teravainen, A., Clark, A. and Shaw, S. (2018) *Literacy and Life Expectancy: An Evidence Review Exploring the Link between Literacy and Life Expectancy in England through Health and Socioeconomic Factors.* National Literacy Trust.

Gill, P., MacLeod, U., Lester, H. and Hegenbarth, A. (2013) *Improving Access to Health Care for Gypsies and Travellers, Homeless People and Sex Workers: An Evidence-Based Commissioning Guide for Clinical Commissioning Groups and Health & Wellbeing Boards.* Available at: www.gypsy-traveller.org/wp-content/uploads/2017/03/RCGP-Social-Inclusion-Commissioning-Guide.pdf (accessed 16 August 2018).

Glasper, A. (2016) Ensuring optimal health care for LGBT patients. *British Journal of Nursing,* 25(13): 768–9.

Gleeson, J., Hemmingway, A. and Rosser, E. (2015) To what extent do health visitors and school nurses have a voice in the policy process? *Community Practitioner,* June: 38–41.

Glen, S. (1998) Emotional and motivational tendencies: the key to quality nursing care? *Nursing Ethics,* 5(1): 36–42.

Goldberg, D.S. (2017) On stigma & health. *The Journal of Law, Medicine & Ethics,* 45(4): 475–83.

Goldberg, D.T. (2015) *Are We All Postracial Yet?* Hoboken, NJ: John Wiley & Sons.

Golden, S., Brown, A., Cauley, J., Chin, M., Gary-Webb, T., Kim, C., et al. (2012) Health disparities in endocrine disorders: biological, clinical, and nonclinical factors – an Endocrine Society scientific statement. *The Journal of Clinical Endocrinology and Metabolism,* 97(9): E1579–639.

Government Equalities Office (2018) *National LGBT Survey Summary Report.* Available at: https://assets.publishing.service.gov.uk/government/uploads/system/uploads/ attachment_data/file/722314/GEO-LGBT-Survey-Report.pdf (accessed 20 August 2019).

Greenfields, M. (2017) Good practice in working with gypsy, traveller and Roma communities. *Primary Health Care,* 27(10): 24–9.

Griffith, J.K. (2009) *The Religious Aspect of Nursing Care.* Available at: https://nursing.ubc. ca/sites/nursing.ubc.ca/files/documents/ReligiousAspectsofNursingCareEEdition.pdf (accessed 2 September 2019).

Green, M.A., Evans, C.R. and Subramanian, S.V. (2017) Can intersectionality theory enrich population health research? *Social Science & Medicine*, 178: 214–26.

Gruer, L., Cézard, G., Clark, E., Douglas, A., Steiner, M., Millard, A., et al. (2016) Life expectancy of different ethnic groups using death records linked to population census data for 4.62 million people in Scotland. *Journal of Epidemiology and Community Health*, 70(12): 1251–4.

Guardian Press Association (2011) *Nurse Jailed for Killing Her Baby by Force-Feeding*. Available at: www.theguardian.com/uk/2011/nov/11/nurse-jailed-baby-force-feeding (accessed 1 August 2018).

Haith, M. (2017) *Understanding Mental Health Practice*. London: Learning Matters.

Hall, S. (ed.) (1997) *Representation: Cultural Representations and Signifying Practices*. London: SAGE.

Haney, A. M. and Rollock, D. (2018) A matter of faith: the role of religion, doubt, and personality in emerging adult mental health. *Psychology of Religion and Spirituality*. Advance online publication.

Hart, P.L. and Moreno, N. (2016) Nurses' perceptions of their cultural competence in caring for diverse patient populations. *Online Journal of Cultural Competence in Nursing and Healthcare*, 6(1): 121–37.

Hastings, A., Bailey, N., Bramley, G. and Gannon, M. (2017) Austerity urbanism in England: the 'regressive redistribution' of local government services and the impact on the poor and marginalised. *Environment and Planning A: Economy and Space*, 49(9): 2007–24.

Hatton, C., Emerson, E., Robertson, J. and Baines, S. (2017) The mental health of British adults with intellectual impairments living in general households. *Journal of Applied Research in Intellectual Disabilities*, 30(1): 188–97.

Haywood, C., Lanzkron, S., Bediako, S., Strouse, J.J., Haythornthwaite, J., Carroll, C.P., et al. (2014) Perceived discrimination, patient trust, and adherence to medical recommendations among persons with sickle cell disease. *Journal of General Internal Medicine*, 29(12): 1657–62.

Healthcare Quality Improvement Partnership (HQIP) (2017) *The Learning Disabilities Mortality Review Annual Report 2017*. Available at: www.hqip.org.uk/resource/the-learning-disabilities-mortality-review-annual-report-2017/ (accessed 20 August 2019).

Health Education England (2018) *Diversity and Inclusion: Our Strategic Framework 2018–2022*. Available at: www.hee.nhs.uk/sites/default/files/documents/Diversity%20and%20Inclusion%20-%20Our%20Strategic%20Framework.pdf (accessed 6 October 2019).

Health Foundation (2018) *What Makes Us Healthy? An Introduction to Social Determinants of Health*. Available at: www.health.org.uk/sites/default/files/What-makes-us-healthy-quick-guide.pdf (accessed 28 September 2019).

Health Protection Agency (HPA) (2013) *Tuberculosis Update*. Available at: https://webarchive.nationalarchives.gov.uk/20140714074616/http://www.hpa.org.uk/webc/HPAwebFile/HPAweb_C/1317138493033 (accessed 21 October 2019).

Heaslip, V. (2015) Caring for people from diverse cultures. *British Journal of Community Nursing*, 20(9): 421.

Henderson, S., Horne, M., Hills, R. and Kendall, E. (2018) Cultural competence in healthcare in the community: a concept analysis. *Health and Social Care in the Community*, 26: 590–603.

Heslop, P., Blair, P., Fleming, P., Hoghton, M., Marriott, A. and Russ, L. (2013) *Confidential Inquiry into Premature Deaths of People with Learning Disabilities (CIPOLD)*. Bristol: Norah Fry Research Centre.

HM Government (2013) *Equality Act 2010: Guidance*. Available at: www.gov.uk/guidance/equality-act-2010-guidance (accessed 5 September 2019).

HM Government (2015) *Working Together to Safeguard Children: A Guide to Inter-Agency Working to Safeguard and Promote the Welfare of Children*. Available at: https://assets.publishing.service.gov.uk/government/uploads/system/uploads/attachment_data/file/592101/Working_Together_to_Safeguard_Children_20170213.pdf (accessed 3 June 2018).

HM Government (2016a) *Childhood Obesity: A Plan for Action*. Available at: www.gov.uk/government/publications/childhood-obesity-a-plan-for-action/childhood-obesity-a-plan-for-action (accessed 3 September 2019).

HM Government (2016b) *Ending Violence against Women and Girls: Strategy 2016–2020*. Available at: https://assets.publishing.service.gov.uk/government/uploads/system/uploads/attachment_data/file/522166/VAWG_Strategy_FINAL_PUBLICATION_MASTER_vRB.PDF (accessed 4 September 2019).

HM Government (2018) *A Connected Society: A Strategy for Tackling Loneliness – Laying the Foundations for Change*. Available at: www.gov.uk/government/publications/a-connected-society-a-strategy-for-tackling-loneliness (accessed 21 October 2019).

HM Treasury (2015) *Soft Drinks Industry Levy Comes into Effect*. Available at: www.gov.uk/government/news/soft-drinks-industry-levy-comes-into-effect (accessed 4 September 2019).

Holland, K. (2018) *Cultural Awareness in Nursing and Health Care: An Introductory Text* (3rd edn). London: Routledge.

Holland, L. and Ousey, K. (2011) Inclusion or exclusion: recruiting black and minority ethnic community individuals as simulated patients. *Ethnicity and Inequalities in Health and Social Care*, 4(2): 81–90.

Holm, A.L., Gorosh, M.R., Brady, M. and White-Perkins, D. (2017) Recognizing privilege and bias: an interactive exercise to expand health care providers' personal awareness. *Academic Medicine*, 92(3): 360–4.

Home Office (2013) *Diversity Strategy 2013–2016: Making the Most of Our Diversity*. Available at: https://assets.publishing.service.gov.uk/government/uploads/system/uploads/attachment_data/file/226459/E_D_Strategy_report_v3.PDF (accessed 28 September 2019).

Hordern, J. (2016) Religion and culture. *Medicine*, 44(10): 589–92.

Huber, M., Knottnerus, J.A., Green, L., van der Horst, H., Jadad, A.R., Kromhout, D., et al. (2011) How should we define health? *BMJ*, 343: d4163.

International Diabetes Federation (2017) *IDF Diabetes Atlas* (8th edn). Available at: www. diabetesatlas.org (accessed 3 September 2019).

Jack, K. and Smith, A. (2007) Promoting self-awareness in nurses to improve nursing practice. *Nursing Standard*, 21(32): 47–52.

Jandt, F.E. and Jandt, F.E. (2018) *An Introduction to Intercultural Communication: Identities in a Global Community* (9th edn). Thousand Oaks, CA: SAGE.

Jasper, M. (2003) *Beginning Reflective Practice*. Cheltenham: Nelson Thomas.

Jehovah's Witnesses (2018) *Information on Blood Transfusion Beliefs*. Available at: www. jw.org/en/search/?q=blood+transfusion (accessed 23 August 2018).

Jhita, T., Petrou, S., Gumber, A., Szczepura, A., Raymond, N.T. and Bellary, S. (2014) Ethnic differences in health-related quality of life for patients with Type 2 diabetes. *Health and Quality of Life Outcomes*, 12(83): 83–92.

Jirwe, M., Gerrish, K. and Emami, A. (2006) The theoretical framework of cultural competence. *Journal of Multicultural Nursing and Health*, September: 6–16.

Johl, N., Patterson, T. and Pearson, L. (2016) What do we know about the attitudes, experiences and needs of black and minority ethnic carers of people with dementia in the United Kingdom? A systematic review of empirical research findings. *Dementia*, 15(4): 721–42.

Jonassaint, C.R., Jones, V.L., Leong, S. and Frierson, G.M. (2016) A systematic review of the association between depression and health care utilization in children and adults with sickle cell disease. *British Journal of Haematology*, 174(1): 136–47.

Jones, A. and Chinegwundoh, F. (2014) Update on prostate cancer in black men within the UK. *ecancermedicalscience*, 8: 455.

Jorm, A.F. (2000) Mental health literacy: public knowledge and beliefs about mental disorders. *British Journal of Psychiatry*, 177: 396–401.

Jorm, A.F., Korten, A.E., Jacomb, P.A., Christensen, H., Rodgers, B. and Pollitt, P. (1997) Mental health literacy: a survey of the public's ability to recognise mental disorders and their belief about the effectiveness of treatment. *Medical Journal of Australia*, 166: 182–6.

Jurcic, M. (2016) *Working with Victims of Anti-LGBT Hate Crimes: A Practical Handbook*. Available at: www.galop.org.uk/wp-content/uploads/Working-with-Victims-of-Anti% E2%80%93LGBT-Hate-Crimes.pdf (accessed 7 October 2019).

Kane, E. (2014) *Prevalence, Patterns and Possibilities: The Experience of People from Black and Ethnic Minorities with Mental Health Problems in the Criminal Justice System*. Available at: https://3bx16p38bchl32s0e12di03h-wpengine.netdna-ssl.com/wp-content/uploads/ 2014/05/prevalence-patterns-and-possibilities.pdf (accessed 9 December 2019).

Kapur, N. (2015) Unconscious bias harms patients and staff. *BMJ*, 351: h6347.

Khalaf, I.A., Al-Dweik, G., Abu-Snieneh, H., Al-Daken, L., Musallam, R.M., BaniYounis, M., et al. (2018) Nurses' experiences of grief following patient death: a qualitative approach. *Journal of Holistic Nursing*, 36(3): 228–40.

Kirkbride, J.B., Barker, D., Cowden, F., Stamps, R., Yang, M., Jones, P.B., et al. (2008) Psychoses, ethnicity and socio-economic status. *British Journal of Psychiatry*, 193(1): 18–24.

Kline, R. (2014) *The Snowy White Peaks of the NHS: A Survey of Discrimination in Governance and Leadership and the Potential Impact on Patient Care in London and England*. Available at: www.england.nhs.uk/wp-content/uploads/2014/08/edc7-0514.pdf (accessed 2 May 2017).

Kline, R. (2015) *Beyond the Snowy White Peaks of the NHS? Diversity in the NHS*. Available at: https://raceequalityfoundation.org.uk/wp-content/uploads/2018/02/Health-Briefing-39-_Final.pdf (accessed 20 August 2019).

Kmietowicz, Z. (2009) Screening has halved incidence of cervical cancer in UK. *BMJ*, 338: b807.

Knapp, M. (2012) Mental health in an age of austerity. *Evidence-Based Mental Health*, 15(3): 54–5.

Knight, P. (2012) Raising cancer awareness in minority ethnic groups. *Nursing Times*, 108(38): 17–19.

Kourkouta, L. and Papathanasiou, I.V. (2014) Communication in nursing practice. *Mater Socio Medica*, 26(1): 65–7.

Lagisetty, P., Priyadarshini, S., Terrell, S., Hamati, M., Landgraf, J., Chopra, V., et al. (2017) Culturally targeted strategies for diabetes prevention in minority populations: a systematic review and framework. *Diabetes Education*, 43(1): 54–77.

Lamb, V. and Joels, C. (2014) Improving access to health care for homeless people. *Nursing Standard*, 29(6): 45–51.

Landrine, H. and Klonoff, E.A. (2004) Culture change and ethnic-minority health behavior: an operant theory of acculturation. *Journal of Behavioral Medicine*, 27(6): 527–55.

Larsson, P. (2013) The rhetoric/reality gap in social determinants of mental health. *Mental Health Review Journal*, 18(4): 182–93.

Lassiter, J.M., Saleh, L., Grov, C., Starks, T., Ventuneac, A. and Parsons, J.T. (2017) Spirituality and multiple dimensions of religion are associated with mental health in gay and bisexual men: results from the One Thousand Strong cohort. *Psychology of Religion and Spirituality*, 11(4): 408–16.

Latif, Z. (2014) *The Maternal Mental Health of Migrant Women*. Available at: www.better-health.org.uk/sites/default/files/briefings/downloads/Health_Briefing_31_0.pdf (accessed 2 May 2017).

Lea, D.H. (2009) Basic genetics and genomics: a primer for nurses. *OJIN: The Online Journal of Issues in Nursing*, 14(2): 1–11.

Ledger, P. and Bowler, B. (2013) Meeting spiritual needs in mental health care. *Nursing Times*, 109(9): 21–3.

Leininger, M.M. (1988) Leininger's theory of nursing: cultural care diversity and universality. *Nursing Science Quarterly*, 1(4): 152–160.

Lexico (2019a) *Communication*. Available at: www.lexico.com/en/definition/coomunication (accessed 21 September 2019).

Lexico (2019b) *Competent*. Available at: www.lexico.com/en/definition/competent (accessed 21 September 2019).

Lexico (2019c) *Quality*. Available at: www.lexico.com/en/definition/quality (accessed 21 September 2019).

LGBT Foundation (2018) *Let's Talk about It: Cervical Screening for Lesbian, Gay and Bisexual Women*. Available https://lgbt.foundation/news/lets-talk-about-it-cervical-screening-for-lesbian-gay-and-bisexual-women/177 (accessed 4 September 2019)

Lo, S. and Horton, R. (2016) Transgender health: an opportunity for global health equity. *The Lancet*, 388(10042): 316–18.

Lonneman, W. (2015) Teaching strategies to increase cultural awareness in nursing students. *Nurse Educator*, 40(6): 285–8.

Luchenski, S., Magurie, N., Aldridge, R., Hayward, A., Story, A., Perri, P., et al. (2018) What works in inclusion health: overview of effective interventions for marginalised and excluded populations. *The Lancet*, 391(10117): 266–80.

Mabuka-Maroa, J. (2019) Africa needs a heavy dose of investment in genomics research. *The Conversation*. Available at: http://theconversation.com/africa-needs-a-heavy-dose-of-investment-in-genomics-research-114456 (accessed 9 December 2019).

Marlow, L.A.V., Chorley, A.J., Haddrell, J., Ferrer, R. and Waller, J. (2017) Understanding the heterogeneity of cervical cancer screening non-participants: data from a national sample of British women. *European Journal of Cancer*, 80: 30–8.

Marmot, M. (2015) *Fair Society, Healthy Lives: A Strategic Review of Health Inequalities in England Post-2010*. London: UCL.

Marmot, M., Allen, J., Goldblatt, P., Boyce, T., McNeish, D., Grady, M., et al. (2010) *The Marmot Review: Fair Society, Healthy Lives – The Strategic Review of Health Inequalities in England Post-2010*. London: UCL.

MBRRACE-UK (2018) *Mothers and Babies Reducing Risks through Audit and Confidential Enquiries across the UK*. Available at: www.npeu.ox.ac.uk/downloads/files/mbrrace-uk/reports/MBRRACE-UK%20Maternal%20Report%202018%20-%20Web%20Version.pdf (accessed 13 April 2019).

McCarthy, A., Lee, K., Itakura, S. and Muir, D. (2006) Cultural display rules drive eye gazing during thinking. *Journal of Cross-Cultural Psychology*, 37(6): 717–22.

McCarthy, J., Cassidy, I., Graham, M. and Tuohy, D. (2013) Conversations through barriers of language and interpretation. *British Journal of Nursing*, 22(6): 335–9.

McClimens, A., Brewster, J. and Lewis, R. (2014) Recognising and respecting patients' cultural diversity. *Nursing Standard*, 28(28): 45–52.

McConnell, E. (2001) Competence vs. competency. *Nursing Management*, 32(5): 14.

McCormack, B. and McCance, T. (eds) (2016) *Person-Centred Practice in Nursing and Health Care: Theory and Practice*. Hoboken, NJ: John Wiley & Sons.

McCullough, S. (2014) *An Exploration of Political Awareness amongst a Cohort of All Field Students, in One University in Northern Ireland*. Available at: http://pure.qub.ac.uk/portal/files/13229771/Trinity_Dublin_Nov_2014.pptx (accessed 4 September 2019).

McDonald, A. (2016) *A Long and Winding Road: Improving Communication with Patients in the NHS*. Available at: www.mariecurie.org.uk/globalassets/media/documents/policy/campaigns/the-long-and-winding-road.pdf (accessed 29 April 2018).

McManus, S., Meltzer, H., Brugha, T., Bebbington, P., Brugha, T., Coid, J., et al. (2009) Adult psychiatric morbidity in England, 2007: results of a household survey. In S. McManus, H. Meltzer, T. Brugha, et al. (eds), *The NHS Information Centre for Health and Social Care*, London.

McSherry, W. and Jamieson, S. (2011) An online survey of nurses' perceptions of spirituality and spiritual care. *Journal of Clinical Nursing*, 20(11–12): 1757–67.

Meddings, F. and Haith-Cooper, M. (2008) Culture and communication in ethically appropriate care. *Nursing Ethics*, 15: 52–61.

Memon, A., Taylor, K., Mohebati, L.M., Sundin, J., Cooper, M., Scanlon, T., et al. (2016) *Perceived Barriers to Accessing Mental Health Services among Black and Minority Ethnic (BME) Communities: A Qualitative Study in Southeast England*. Available at: https://bmjopen.bmj.com/content/bmjopen/6/11/e012337.full.pdf (accessed 1 July 2018).

Mencap (2013) *Mencap Research: 'Scandal of Avoidable Death' as 1,200 People with a Learning Disability Die Needlessly Every Year in NHS Care*. Available at: www.mencap.org.uk/press-release/mencap-research-scandal-avoidable-death-1200-people-learning-disability-die (accessed 6 October 2019).

Mencap (n.d.) *What Is a Learning Disability?* Available at: www.mencap.org.uk/learning-disability-explained/what-learning-disability (accessed 24 June 2018).

Mendes, A. (2015) Culture and religion in nursing: providing culturally sensitive care. *British Journal of Nursing*, 24(8): 459.

Mental Health Foundation (2016) *Fundamental Facts about Mental Health*. Available at: www.mentalhealth.org.uk/publications/fundamental-facts-about-mental-health-2016 (accessed 30 June 2019).

Mereish, E.H., Liu, M.M. and Helms, J.E. (2012) Effects of discrimination on Chinese, Filipino, and Vietnamese Americans' mental and physical health. *Asian American Journal of Psychology*, 3(2): 91–103.

Metzl, J. (2010) *The Protest Psychosis: How Schizophrenia Became a Black Disease*. Boston, MA: Beacon Press.

Mind (2013) *Mental Health Crisis Care: Commissioning Excellence for BME Groups*. Available at: www.mind.org.uk/media/494422/bme-commissioning-excellence-briefing.pdf (accessed 2 May 2017).

Moffatt, S., Lawson, S., Patterson, R., Holding, E., Dennison, A., Sowden, S., et al. (2016) A qualitative study of the impact of the UK 'bedroom tax'. *Journal of Public Health*, 38(2): 197–205.

Morgan, C., Abdul-Al, R., Lappin, J.M., Jones, P., Fearon, P., Leese, M., et al. (2006) Clinical and social determinants of duration of untreated psychosis in the AESOP first-episode psychosis study. *British Journal of Psychiatry*, 189(5): 446–52.

Moro, T.T., Savage, T.A. and Gehlert, S. (2017) Agency, social and healthcare supports for adults with intellectual disability at the end of life in out-of-home, non-institutional community residences in Western nations: a literature review. *Journal of Applied Research in Intellectual Disabilities*, 30(6): 1045–56.

Murji, K. and Solomos, J. (2015) Conclusion: back to the future. In K. Murji and J. Solomos (eds), *Theories of Race and Ethnicity: Contemporary Debates and Perspectives*. Cambridge: Cambridge University Press.

Murray, R.B. and Zentner, J.B. (1989) *Nursing Concepts for Health Promotion*. London: Prentice Hall.

Myers, J. (2015) Challenges of identifying eczema in darkly pigmented skin. *Nursing Children and Young People*, 27(6): 24–8.

Narrative Inquiry in Bioethics Editors (2014) Introduction: religion in medical and nursing practice. *Narrative Inquiry in Bioethics*, 4(3): 189–90.

National Health Service Act (1946) Available at: www.legislation.gov.uk/ukpga/1946/81/pdfs/ukpga_19460081_en.pdf (accessed 6 October 2019).

National Literacy Trust (2017) *Adult Literacy*. Available at: https://literacytrust.org.uk/parents-and-families/adult-literacy/ (accessed 7 April 2018).

National Service Framework for Mental Health (1999) *Mental Health*. Available at: https://assets.publishing.service.gov.uk/government/uploads/system/uploads/attachment_data/file/198051/National_Service_Framework_for_Mental_Health.pdf (accessed 29 June 2018).

Nazroo, J. (n.d.) *Ethnic Inequalities in Health: Addressing a Significant Gap in Current Evidence and Policy*. Available at: www.thebritishacademy.ac.uk/sites/default/files/James%20Y.%20Nazroo%20-%20Ethnic%20Inequalities%20in%20Health%20-%20Addressing%20a%20Significant%20Gap%20in%20Current%20Evidence.pdf (accessed 21 October 2019).

Nelson, T.D. (2009) *Handbook of Prejudice, Stereotyping, and Discrimination*. New York: Psychology Press.

Nelson, T.D. (2015) *Handbook of Prejudice, Stereotyping, and Discrimination* (2nd edn). London: Routledge.

NHS (2016) *NHS Workforce Race Equality Standard: 2015 Data Analysis Report for NHS Trusts*. Available at: www.england.nhs.uk/wp-content/uploads/2014/10/WRES-Data-Analysis-Report.pdf (accessed 2 May 2017).

NHS (2019) *Breast Cancer Screening*. Available at: www.nhs.uk/conditions/breast-cancer-screening/ (accessed 29 August 2019).

NHS Digital (2018) *Statistics on Care of People with Learning Disabilities*. Available at: https://digital.nhs.uk/news-and-events/latest-news/statistics-for-care-of-people-with-learning-difficulties (accessed 29 August 2019).

NHS England (2012) *Our Culture of Compassionate Care: Creating a Vision for Nurses, Midwives and Care Staff.* Available at: www.england.nhs.uk/wp-content/uploads/2012/12/6c-visual.pdf (accessed 24 April 2018).

NHS England (2014a) *Action for Diabetes.* Available at: www.england.nhs.uk/rightcare/wp-content/uploads/sites/40/2016/08/act-for-diabetes-31-01.pdf (accessed 4 September 2019).

NHS England (2014b) *Five Year Forward View.* Available at: www.england.nhs.uk/wp-content/uploads/2014/10/5yfv-web.pdf (accessed 4 September 2019).

NHS England (2015) *Introducing the 6Cs.* Available at: https://www.england.nhs.uk/6cs/wp-content/uploads/sites/25/2015/03/introducing-the-6cs.pdf (accessed 13 November 2019).

NHS England (2016a) *Five Year Forward View for Mental Health.* Available at: www.england.nhs.uk/wp-content/uploads/2016/02/Mental-Health-Taskforce-FYFV-final.pdf (accessed 4 September 2019).

NHS England (2016b) *Leading Change, Adding Value: A Framework for Nursing, Midwifery and Care Staff.* Available at: www.england.nhs.uk/wp-content/uploads/2016/05/nursing-framework.pdf (accessed 16 August 2018).

NHS Health and Social Care Information Centre (2005) *Health Survey for England 2004: The Health of Minority Ethnic Groups.* Available at: https://files.digital.nhs.uk/publicationimport/pub01xxx/pub01209/heal-surv-hea-eth-min-hea-tab-eng-2004-rep.pdf (accessed 3 September 2019).

NHS Improvement (2018) *The Learning Disability Improvement Standards for NHS Trusts.* Available at: https://improvement.nhs.uk/resources/learning-disability-improvement-standards-nhs-trusts/ (accessed 2 December 2018).

NHS Scotland (2019) *Scottish Palliative Care Guidelines: Patient and Family Focus.* Available at: www.palliativecareguidelines.scot.nhs.uk/guidelines/about-the-guidelines/patient-and-family-focus.aspx (accessed 13 October 2019).

NHS Scotland Chaplaincy Services (2007) *Standards for NHS Scotland Chaplaincy Services.* Available at: www.nes.scot.nhs.uk/media/290156/chaplaincy__standards_final_version.pdf (accessed 13 October 2019).

NICE (2012) *Patient Experience in Adult NHS Services.* Available at: www.nice.org.uk/guidance/qs15 (accessed 12 August 2018).

Nordenfelt, L. (2007) The concepts of health and illness revisited. *Medicine, Health Care and Philosophy*, 10(1): 5–10.

Norouzinia, R., Aghabarari, M., Shiri, M., Karimi, M. and Samami, E. (2016) Communication barriers perceived by nurses and patients. *Global Journal of Health Science*, 8(6): 65–74.

NSC NHS Strategic Health Authority (2003) *Independent Inquiry into the Death of David Bennett: An Independent Inquiry Set Up under HSG (94)27.* Available at: www.rbmind.org/DocumentLibrary/DavidBennettEquiry.pdf (accessed 2 May 2017).

Nursing and Midwifery Council (NMC) (2004) *Standards of Proficiency for Specialist Community Public Health Nurses.* Available at: www.nmc.org.uk/globalassets/site documents/standards/nmc-standards-of-proficiency-for-specialist-community-public-health-nurses.pdf (accessed 3 September 2019).

Nursing and Midwifery Council (NMC) (2012) *Conduct and Competence Committee: Substantive Hearing Case Gloria Dwomoh.* Available at: www.nmc.org.uk/globalassets/sitedocuments/ftpoutcomes/2012/october/reasons-dwomoh-cccsh-29808-20121022.pdf (accessed 10 August 2018).

Nursing and Midwifery Council (NMC) (2015) *The Code: Professional Standards of Practice and Behaviour for Nurses and Midwives.* Available at: www.nmc.org.uk/globalassets/site documents/nmc-publications/nmc-code.pdf (accessed 1 July 2018).

Nursing and Midwifery Council (NMC) (2017) *Enabling Professionalism.* Available at: www.nmc.org.uk/globalassets/sitedocuments/other-publications/enabling-professionalism.pdf (accessed 22 August 2018).

Nursing and Midwifery Council (NMC) (2018) *Future Nurse: Standards of Proficiency for Registered Nurses.* Available at: www.nmc.org.uk/globalassets/sitedocuments/education-standards/future-nurse-proficiencies.pdf (accessed 25 June 2018).

Nursing and Midwifery Council (NMC) (2019) *Concerns, Complaints and Referrals.* Available at: www.nmc.org.uk/concerns-nurses-midwives/concerns-complaints-and-referrals/ (accessed 24 October 2019).

Nutbeam, D. (2004) Getting evidence into policy and practice to address health inequalities. *Health Promotion International,* 19(2): 137–40.

Nutbeam, D. (2008) The evolving concept of health literacy. *Social Science & Medicine,* 67: 2072–8.

Nyatanga, B. (2018) Cultural competence in palliative care and a world of multiculturalism. *British Journal of Community Nursing,* 23(6): 307.

O'Connell, M.B., Korner, E.J., Rickles, N.M. and Sias, J.J. (2007) Cultural competence in health care and its implications for pharmacy. Part 1: overview of key concepts in Perez-Bret, E. Altisent, R. and Rocafort, J. (2016) Definition of compassion in healthcare: a systematic literature review. *International Journal of Palliative Nursing,* 22(12): 599–606.

Office for National Statistics (ONS) (2012) *Religion in England and Wales 2011.* Available at: www.ons.gov.uk/peoplepopulationandcommunity/culturalidentity/religion/articles/religioninenglandandwales2011/2012-12-11#targetText=In%20the%202011%20Census%2C%20Christianity,per%20cent%20of%20the%20population (accessed 13 October 2019).

Office for National Statistics (ONS) (2013) *2011 Census: Detailed Characteristics for England and Wales, March 2011.* Available at: www.ons.gov.uk/peoplepopulationandcommunity/populationandmigration/populationestimates/bulletins/2011census/2013-05-16 (accessed 6 October 2019).

Office for National Statistics (ONS) (2014) *2011 Census Analysis: What Does the 2011 Census Tell Us about the Characteristics of Gypsy or Irish Travellers in England and Wales?*

Available at: www.ons.gov.uk/peoplepopulationandcommunity/culturalidentity/ethnicity/datasets/2011censusanalysiswhatdoesthe2011censustellusaboutthecharacteristicsofgypsyoririshtravellersinenglandandwales (accessed 1 July 2018).

Office for National Statistics (ONS) (2015) *How Has Life Expectancy Changed over Time?* Available at: www.ons.gov.uk/peoplepopulationandcommunity/birthsdeaths andmarriages/lifeexpectancies/articles/howhaslifeexpectancychangedovertime/2015-09-09 (accessed 3 September 2019).

Office for National Statistics (ONS) (2016) *Sexual Identity, UK: 2016.* Available at: www.ons.gov.uk/peoplepopulationandcommunity/culturalidentity/sexuality/bulletins/sexualidentityuk/2016 (accessed 3 September 2019).

Office for National Statistics (ONS) (2017) *National Life Tables, UK: 2014 to 2016.* Available at: www.ons.gov.uk/peoplepopulationandcommunity/birthsdeathsand-marriages/lifeexpectancies/bulletins/nationallifetablesunitedkingdom/2014to2016 (accessed 29 August 2019).

Office for National Statistics (ONS) (2018) *Overview of the UK Population: November 2018.* Available at: www.ons.gov.uk/peoplepopulationandcommunity/populationandmigration/populationestimates/articles/overviewoftheukpopulation/november2018 (accessed 3 September 2019).

Office for National Statistics (ONS) (2019a) *Overview of the UK Population: August 2019.* Available at: www.ons.gov.uk/peoplepopulationandcommunity/populationandmigration/populationestimates/articles/overviewoftheukpopulation/august2019/previous/v1 (accessed 29 September 2019).

Office for National Statistics (ONS) (2019b) *Population Estimates for the UK, England and Wales, Scotland and Northern Ireland: Mid-2018.* Available at: www.ons.gov.uk/peoplepopu lationandcommunity/populationandmigration/populationestimates/bulletins/annual midyearpopulationestimates/mid2018 (accessed 5 October 2019).

Office for National Statistics (ONS) (2019c) *Sexual Orientation, UK: 2017.* Available at: www.ons.gov.uk/peoplepopulationandcommunity/culturalidentity/sexuality/bulletins/sexualidentityuk/2017 (accessed 5 October 2019).

Office of Disease Prevention and Health Promotion (ODPHP) (n.d.) *Lesbian, Gay, Bisexual, and Transgender Health.* Available at: www.healthypeople.gov/2020/topics-objectives/topic/lesbian-gay-bisexual-and-transgender-health (accessed 3 April 2019).

O'Hagan, K. (2001) *Cultural Competence in the Caring Professions.* London: Jessica Kingsley.

Oman, D. (2011) Spiritual practice, health promotion, and the elusive soul: perspectives from public health. *Pastoral Psychology*, 60(6): 897–906.

Oman, D. and Thoresen, C.E. (2005) Do religion and spirituality influence health? In R.F. Paloutzian and C.L. Park (eds), *Handbook of the Psychology of Religion and Spirituality.* New York: Guilford Press.

O'Neill, J., Tabish, H., Welch, V., Petticrew, M., Pottie, K., Clarke, M., et al. (2014) Applying an equity lens to interventions: using PROGRESS ensures consideration of socially stratifying factors to illuminate inequities in health. *Journal of Clinical Epidemiology*, 67(1): 56–64.

Oozageer Gunowa, N., Hutchinson, M., Brooke, J. and Jackson, D. (2018) Pressure injuries in people with darker skin tones: a literature review. *Journal of Clinical Nursing*, 27(17–18): 3266–75.

Osborne, H. (2013) *Health Literacy from A to Z: Practical Ways to Communicate Your Health Message* (2nd edn). Burlington, MA: Jones & Bartlett Learning.

Papadopoulos, I. (2006) *Transcultural Health and Social Care: Development of Culturally Competent Practitioners*. Edinburgh: Churchill Livingstone.

Papadopoulos, I. (2014) *The Papadopoulos Model for Developing Culturally Competent Compassion in Healthcare Professionals*. Available at: www.youtube.com/watch?v=zjKzO94TevA (accessed 3 February 2019).

Papadopoulos, I. (2018) *Culturally Competent Compassion: A Guide for Healthcare Students and Practitioners*. London: Routledge.

Papadopoulos, I. and Pezella, A. (2015) A snapshot review of culturally competent compassion as addressed in selected mental health textbooks for undergraduate nursing students. *Journal of Compassionate Healthcare*, 2(3). Available at: https://jcompassionatehc.biomedcentral.com/track/pdf/10.1186/s40639-015-0012-5 (accessed 21 October 2019).

Papadopoulos, I., Tilki, M. and Taylor, G. (1998) *Transcultural Care: A Guide for Health Care Professionals*. Dinton: Quay Publications.

Parekh, B. (2000) *Rethinking Multiculturalism: Cultural Diversity and Political Theory*. London: Macmillan.

Parikh, N.S., Parker, R.M., Nurss, J., Baker, D.W. and Williams, M.V. (1996) Shame and health literacy: the unspoken connection. *Patient Education and Counselling*, 27(1): 33–9.

Parliament UK (2019) *What We Know about Inequalities Facing Gypsy, Roma and Traveller Communities*. Available at: https://publications.parliament.uk/pa/cm201719/cmselect/cmwomeq/360/report-files/36005.htm#targetText=42%20per%20cent%20of%20English,the%20non%2DTraveller%20community.22 (accessed 19 September 2019).

Pavord, E. and Donnelly, E. (2015) *Communication and Interpersonal Skills*. Banbury: Lantern.

Peacock, S. and Patel, S. (2008) Cultural influences on pain. *Reviews in Pain*, 1(2): 6–8.

Peate, I. (2016) Transgender equality. *British Journal of Nursing*, 25(5): 239.

Pentaris, P. (2018) The marginalization of religion in end of life care: signs of micro-aggression? *International Journal of Human Rights in Healthcare*, 11(2): 116–28.

Peplau, H.E. (1987) Interpersonal constructs for nursing practice. *Nurse Education Today*, 7: 201–8.

Perez-Bret, E., Altisent, R. and Rocafort, J. (2016) Definition of compassion in healthcare: a systematic literature review. *International Journal of Palliative Nursing*, 22(12): 599–606.

Pesut, B. (2016) There be dragons: effects of unexplored religion on nurses' competence in spiritual care. *Nursing inquiry*, 23(3): 191–9.

Phillips, G., Lifford, K., Edwards, A., Poolman, M. and Joseph-Williams, N. (2019) Do published patient decision aids for end-of-life care address patients' decision-making needs? A systematic review and critical appraisal. *Palliative Medicine*, 33(8): 985–1002.

Price, B. (2017) Improving nurses' level of reflection. *Nursing Standard*, 32(1): 52–61.

Prins, H., Backer-Hoist, T., Francis, E., et al. (eds) (1993) *Report of the Committee of Inquiry into the Death in Broadmoor Hospital of Orville Blackwood and a Review of the Deaths of Two Other Afro-Caribbean Patients: Big, Black and Dangerous?* London: Special Hospitals Service Authority.

Prostate Cancer UK (2014) *Behind the Numbers: Getting Statistics Right for Men with Prostate Cancer.* Available at: https://prostatecanceruk.org/about-us/news-and-views/blog-old/2014/9/behind-the-numbers-getting-statistics-right-for-men-with-prostate-cancer (accessed 4 September 2019).

Prostate Cancer UK (2016) *Consensus Statements on PSA Testing in Asymptomatic Men in the UK: Information for Healthcare Professionals.* Available at: https://prostatecanceruk.org/about-us/what-we-think-and-do/consensus-on-psa-testing (accessed 4 September 2019).

Public Health England (PHE) (2014a) *Protecting Your Child against Flu: Information for Parents – Flu Immunisation in England.* Available at: https://assets.publishing.service.gov.uk/government/uploads/system/uploads/attachment_data/file/714954/PHE_Protecting_Child_Flu_DL_leaflet.pdf (accessed 12 August 2018).

Public Health England (PHE) (2014b) *Vaccines and Porcine Gelatine.* Available at: https://assets.publishing.service.gov.uk/government/uploads/system/uploads/attachment_data/file/824013/PHE_vaccines_porcine_gelatine.pdf (accessed 21 September 2019).

Public Health England (PHE) (2014c) *The Children's Flu Vaccination Programme, the Nasal Flu Vaccine Fluenz and Porcine Gelatine: Your Questions Answered.* Available at: https://assets.publishing.service.gov.uk/government/uploads/system/uploads/attachment_data/file/386842/2902998_PHE_FluPorcine_QAforParents_FINAL_CT.pdf (accessed 15 August 2018).

Public Health England (PHE) (2014d) *From Evidence to Action: Opportunities to Protect and Improve the Nation's Health.* Available at: https://assets.publishing.service.gov.uk/government/uploads/system/uploads/attachment_data/file/366852/PHE_Priorities.pdf (accessed 21 October 2019).

Public Health England (PHE) (2014e) *Tuberculosis in the UK: 2014 Report.* Available at: https://assets.publishing.service.gov.uk/government/uploads/system/uploads/attachment_data/file/360335/TB_Annual_report__4_0_300914.pdf (accessed 21 October 2019)

Public Health England (PHE) (2015a) *Collaborative TB Strategy for England: 2015 to 2020.* Available at: https://assets.publishing.service.gov.uk/government/uploads/system/uploads/attachment_data/file/403231/Collaborative_TB_Strategy_for_England_2015_2020_.pdf (accessed 3 September 2019).

Public Health England (PHE) (2015b) *Improving Health Literacy to Reduce Health Inequalities.* Available at: https://assets.publishing.service.gov.uk/government/uploads/system/uploads/attachment_data/file/460709/4a_Health_Literacy-Full.pdf (accessed 26April 2018).

Public Health England (PHE) (2016) *Learning Disabilities Observatory: People with Learning Disabilities in England 2015 – Main Report.* Available at: https://assets.publishing. service.gov.uk/government/uploads/system/uploads/attachment_data/file/613182/ PWLDIE_2015_main_report_NB090517.pdf (accessed 21 October 2019).

Public Health England (PHE) (2017a) *Psychosocial Pathways and Health Incomes: Informing Action on Health Inequalities.* Available at: www.instituteofhealthequity.org/ resources-reports/psychosocial-pathways-and-health-outcomes-informing-action-on-health-inequalities/psychosocial-pathways-and-health-outcomes.pdf (accessed 5 September 2019).

Public Health England (2017b) *Seasonal Flu Guidance for Healthcare Staff and Custodial Staff in Prisons and Other Prescribed Places of Detention for Adults in England: Preventing and Responding to Seasonal Flu Cases or Outbreaks.* Available at: https://assets.publishing. service.gov.uk/government/uploads/system/uploads/attachment_data/file/648192/ Preventing_and_responding_to_seasonal_flu_cases_or_outbreaks_in_prisons_2017_ to_2018.pdf (accessed 4 September 2019).

Public Health England (2017c) *Supporting Women with Learning Disabilities to Access Cervical Screening.* Available at: www.gov.uk/government/publications/cervical-screening-supporting-women-with-learning-disabilities/supporting-women-with-learning-disabilities-to-access-cervical-screening (accessed 4 September 2019).

Public Health England (PHE) (2017d) *Tackling Tuberculosis in Under-Served Populations: A Resource for TB Control Boards and Their Partners.* Available at: www.gov.uk/government/ publications/tackling-tuberculosis-in-under-served-populations (accessed 21 October 2019).

Public Health England (PHE) (2017e) *Reducing Health Inequalities: System, Scale and Sustainability.* Available at: https://assets.publishing.service.gov.uk/government/uploads/ system/uploads/attachment_data/file/731682/Reducing_health_inequalities_system_ scale_and_sustainability.pdf (accessed 6 October 2019).

Public Health England (PHE) (2019) *Having a Smear Test: An Easy Guide about a Health Test for Women Aged 25 to 64.* Available at: https://assets.publishing.service.gov.uk/ government/uploads/system/uploads/attachment_data/file/790791/CSP05_an_easy_ guide_to_cervical_screening.pdf (accessed 21 October 2019).

Purnell, L. (2016) Are we really measuring cultural competence? *Nursing Science Quarterly,* 29(2): 124–7.

Qassem, T., Bebbington, P., Spiers, N., McManus, S., Jenkins, R. and Dein, S. (2015) Prevalence of psychosis in black ethnic minorities in Britain: analysis based on three national surveys. *Social Psychiatry and Psychiatric Epidemiology,* 50(7): 1057–64.

Queens Nursing Institute (2015) *Assessing the Health of People Who Are Homeless: Guidance with Health Assessment Tool (2015).* Available at: www.qni.org.uk/wp-content/ uploads/2016/10/HAT_final_web.pdf (accessed 4 September 2019).

Quinn, B. (2018) Spiritual care is not as complex as we may think. *Nursing Standard,* 33(9): 69–70.

Race Equality Foundation (2015) *Better Practice in Mental Health for Black and Minority Ethnic Communities.* Available at: http://raceequalityfoundation.org.uk/wp-content/ uploads/2018/10/Better-practice-in-mental-health.pdf (accessed 2 May 2017).

Ramezani, M., Ahmadi, F., Mohammadi, E. and Kazemnejad, A. (2014) Spiritual care in nursing: a concept analysis. *International Nursing Review*, 61(2): 211–19.

Rauf, A. (2011) *Caring for Dementia: Exploring Good Practice on Supporting South Asian Carers.* Bradford Metropolitan District Council.

Rehman, H. and Owen, D. (2013) *Mental Health Survey of Ethnic Minorities.* Ethnos Research and Consultancy.

Reimer-Kirkham, S. (2014) Nursing research on religion and spirituality through a social justice lens. *Advances in Nursing Science*, 37(3): 249–57.

Reus-Pons, M., Kibele, E.U.B. and Janssen, F. (2017) Differences in healthy life expectancy between older migrants and non-migrants in three European countries over time. *International Journal of Public Health*, 62(5): 531–40.

Reynolds, F., Stanistreet, D. and Elton, P. (2008) Women with learning disabilities and access to cervical screening: retrospective cohort study using case control methods. *BMC Public Health*, 8: 30.

Richardson, B. (2017) *Clinical Skills for Nursing Practice.* London: Routledge.

Richman, L.S. and Hatzenbuehler, M.L. (2014) A multilevel analysis of stigma and health: implications for research and policy. *Health and Wellbeing*, 1(1): 213–21.

Rickard, W. and Donkin, A. (2018) *A Fair, Supportive Society: Summary Report – Institute of Health Equity.* London: UCL.

Robertson, J., Hatton, C., Baines, S. and Emerson, E. (2015) Systematic reviews of the health or health care of people with intellectual disabilities: a systematic review to identify gaps in the evidence base. *Journal of Applied Research in Intellectual Disabilities*, 28(6): 455–523.

Robinson, F. (2019) Caring for LGBT patients in the NHS. *BMJ*, 366: l5374.

Rogers, M. and Wattis, J. (2015) Spirituality in nursing practice. *Nursing Standard*, 29(39): 51–7.

Roper, N., Logan, W. and Tierney, A.J. (2002) *The Roper–Logan–Tierney Model of Nursing: Based on Activities of Living* (3rd edn). London: Elsevier.

Royal College of General Practitioners (RCGP) (2013) *Improving Access to Health Care for Gypsies and Travellers, Homeless People and Sex Workers.* University of Birmingham. Available at: https://www.healthysuffolk.org.uk/uploads/RCGP-Social-Inclusion-Commissioning-Guide.pdf (accessed 9 December 2019).

Royal College of General Practitioners (RCGP) (2014) *Health Literacy Report from an RCGP-Led Health Literacy Workshop.*

Royal College of Nursing (RCN) (2003) *Review of the Year and Summary Accounts 2002/2003.* Available at: www.rcn.org.uk/-/media/royal-college-of-nursing/documents/publications/2003/pub-002059.pdf (accessed 4 September 2019).

Royal College of Nursing (RCN) (2010) *Principles of Nursing Practice.* Available at: www.rcn.org.uk/professional-development/principles-of-nursing-practice (accessed 10 August 2018).

Royal College of Nursing (RCN) (2011) *Spiritual Survey 2010.* Available at: www.rcn.org.uk/professional-development/publications/pub-003861 (accessed 13 August 2019).

Royal College of Nursing (RCN) (2016a) *Caring for Lesbian, Gay, Bisexual or Trans Clients or Patients: Guide for Nurses and Health Care Support Workers on Next of Kin Issues.* Available at: www.rcn.org.uk/professional-development/publications/pub-005592 (accessed 28 September 2019).

Royal College of Nursing (RCN) (2016b) *Culture and Spirituality.* Available at: https://rcni.com/hosted-content/rcn/fundamentals-of-end-of-life-care/culture-and-spirituality (accessed 2 September 2019).

Royal College of Nursing (RCN) (2017a) *Helping Students Get the Best from Their Practice Placements: A Royal College of Nursing Toolkit.* Available at: www.rcn.org.uk/professional-development/publications/pub-006035 (accessed 31 January 2019).

Royal College of Nursing (RCN) (2017b) *The Needs of People with Learning Disabilities: What Pre-Registration Nurses Should Know.* Available at: https://www.rcn.org.uk/professional-development/publications/pub-005769 (accessed 9 December 2019).

Sanford, M. and Michon, N.J. (2019) Buddhist chaplaincy. In *Oxford Research Encyclopedia of Religion.*

Sartori, P. (2010) Spirituality 1: should spirituality and religious beliefs be part of patient care? *Nursing Times,* 106(28): 14–17.

Scadding, J. and Sweeney, S. (2018) *Digital Exclusion in Gypsy and Roma Travellers in the United Kingdom.* Available at: www.gypsy-traveller.org/wp-content/uploads/2018/09/Digital-Inclusion-in-Gypsy-and-Traveller-communities-FINAL-1.pdf (accessed 4 November 2018).

Schultz, P.L. and Baker, J. (2017) Teaching strategies to increase nursing student acceptance and management of unconscious bias. *Journal of Nursing Education,* 56(11): 692–6.

Seidler, Z.E., Dawes, A.J., Rice, S.M., Oliffe, J.L. and Dhillon, H.M. (2016) The role of masculinity in men's help-seeking for depression: a systematic review. *Clinical Psychology Review,* 49: 106–18.

Setta, S.M. and Shemie, S.D. (2015) An explanation and analysis of how world religions formulate their ethical decisions on withdrawing treatment and determining death. *Philosophy, Ethics, and Humanities in Medicine,* 10(1): 6.

Sharma, M., Nazareth, I. and Petersen, I. (2016) Trends in incidence, prevalence and prescribing in Type 2 diabetes mellitus between 2000 and 2013 in primary care: a retrospective cohort study. *BMJ Open,* 6: e010210.

Shelter (2017) *More Than 300,000 People in Britain Homeless Today.* Available at: https://england.shelter.org.uk/media/press_releases/articles/more_than_300,000_people_in_britain_homeless_today (accessed 3 September 2019).

Sivaprasad, S., Gupta, B., Gulliford, M., Dodhia, H., Mohamed, M., Nagi, D., et al. (2012) Ethnic variations in the prevalence of diabetic retinopathy in people with diabetes attending screening in the UK (DRIVE UK). *PLOS One,* 7(3): e32182.

Solomos, J. (2003) *Race and Racism in Britain* (3rd edn). Macmillan International Higher Education.

Sommers, M.S. (2011) Color awareness: a must for patient assessment. *American Nurse Today*, 6(1): 6.

Spanakis, E. and Golden, S. (2013) Race/ethnic differences in diabetes and diabetic complications. *Current Diabetic Reviews*, 13(6): 814–23.

Spritzer, J. (2003) *Caring for Jewish Patients.* Oxford: Radcliffe Publishing.

Srivastava, R. (2003) *The Healthcare's Professional's Guide to Clinical Cultural Competence.* Canada: Mosby.

Stangor, C. (2009) The study of stereotyping, prejudice and discrimination within social psychology: a quick history of theory and research. In T.D. Nelson (ed.), *Handbook of Prejudice, Stereotyping and Discrimination.* London: Routledge.

Starnino, V.R. (2016) Conceptualizing spirituality and religion for mental health practice: perspectives of consumers with serious mental illness. *Families in Society*, 97(4): 295–304.

Story, A., Aldridge, R., Gray, T., Burridge, S. and Hayward, A. (2014) Influenza vaccination, inverse care and homelessness: cross-sectional survey of eligibility and uptake during the 2011/12 season in London. *BMC Public Health*, 14(1): 44.

Sturmberg, J. (2014) Emergent properties define the subjective nature of health and disease. *Journal of Public Health Policy*, 35(3): 414–19.

Sullivan, R. (2014) A 5-year retrospective study of descriptors associated with identification of stage I and suspected deep tissue pressure ulcers in persons with darkly pigmented skin. *Wounds: A Compendium of Clinical Research and Practice*, 26(12): 351–9.

Sunak, R. and Rajeswaran, S. (2014) *A Portrait of Modern Britain.* Available at: https://policyexchange.org.uk/wp-content/uploads/2016/09/a-portrait-of-modern-britain.pdf (accessed 9 December 2019).

Taylor, G. (2015) Exposure to other fields of nursing. In D. Burns (ed.), *Foundations of Adult Nursing.* London: SAGE.

Taylor, S.P., Nicolle, C. and Maguire, M. (2013) Cross-cultural communication barriers in health care. *Nursing Standard*, 27(31): 35–43.

The Evidence Centre (2013) *Content Analysis of 'Patient Opinion' Website Stories about Nurse Attitudes and Behaviours.* Available at: www.careopinion.org.uk/resources/blog-resources/1-files/rcn-professional-attitudes-behaviours-patient-opinion-stories-report.pdf (accessed 11 August 2018).

Timmins, F. and Caldeira, S. (2017a) Assessing the spiritual needs of patients. *Nursing Standard*, 31(29): 47–53.

Timmins, F. and Caldeira, S. (2017b) Understanding spirituality and spiritual care in nursing. *Nursing Standard*, 31(22): 50–7.

Tran, L., Wong, C., Leung, J. and Lam, J. (2008) *Community Engagement Project: The National Institute for Mental Health in England Community Engagement Programme 20067/08. Report of the Community Led Research Project Focussing on the Mental Health Service Needs of*

Chinese Elders in Westminster, Kensington & Chelsea and Brent. London: Chinese National Healthy Living Centre.

Trueland, J. (2014) Eating for health. *Nursing Standard,* 29(5): 24–5.

Truswell, D. (2013) Black, Asian and Minority Ethnic Communities and Dementia: Where Are We Now? *Better Health Briefing,* 30. Available at: https://www.gmmh.nhs.uk/download.cfm?doc=docm93jijm4n898.pdf&ver=1681 (accessed 9 December 2019).

Tuffrey-Wijne, I., Giatras, N., Goulding, L., Abraham, E., Fenwick, L., Edwards, C., et al. (2013) *Identifying the Factors Affecting the Implementation of Strategies to Promote a Safer Environment for Patients with Learning Disabilities in NHS Hospitals: A Mixed Methods Study.* Available at: www.journalslibrary.nihr.ac.uk/hsdr/hsdr01130/#/abstract (accessed 29 April 2018).

Tuffrey-Wijne, I., McLaughlin, D., Curfs, L., Dusart, A., Hoenger, C., McEnhill, L., et al. (2016) Defining consensus norms for palliative care of people with intellectual disabilities in Europe, using Delphi methods: a White Paper from the European Association of Palliative Care. *Palliative Medicine,* 30(5): 446–55.

Turner, N., Hastings, J.F. and Neighbors, H.W. (2018) Mental health care treatment seeking among African Americans and Caribbean blacks: what is the role of religiosity/spirituality? *Aging & Mental Health,* 23(7): 905–11.

Twyman, L., Bonevski, B., Paul, C. and Bryant, J. (2014) Perceived barriers to smoking cessation in selected vulnerable groups: a systematic review of the qualitative and quantitative literature. *BMJ Open,* 4: e006414.

UCL Institute of Health Inequality (2010) *Fair Society, Healthier Lives: Marmot Review.* Available at: www.instituteofhealthequity.org/resources-reports/fair-society-healthy-lives-the-marmot-review/fair-society-healthy-lives-full-report-pdf.pdf (accessed 4 September 2019).

Underwood, S.M. (2006) Culture, diversity, and health: responding to the queries of inquisitive minds. *Journal of Nursing Education,* 45(7): 281–6.

University of Bristol (2018) *The Learning Disabilities Mortality Review (LeDeR) Programme: Annual Report 2017.* Available at: www.bristol.ac.uk/media-library/sites/sps/leder/leder_annual_report_2016-2017.pdf (accessed 5 October 2019).

University of Bristol (2019) *The Learning Disability Mortality Review (LeDeR) Programme: Annual Report 2018.* Available at: www.bristol.ac.uk/media-library/sites/sps/leder/LeDeR_Annual_Report_2018%20published%20May%202019.pdf (accessed 7 October 2019).

van Os, J. (2012) Psychotic experiences: disadvantaged and different from the norm. *British Journal of Psychiatry,* 201: 258–9.

Venkatasalu, M.R. (2017) Let him not be alone: perspectives of older British South Asian minority ethnic patients on dying in acute hospitals. *International Journal of Palliative Nursing,* 23(9): 432–9.

Vertovec, S. (2011) The cultural politics of nation and migration. *Annual Review of Anthropology,* 40: 241–56.

Viruell-Fuentes, E.A., Miranda, P.Y. and Abdulrahim, S. (2012) More than culture: structural racism, intersectionality theory, and immigrant health. *Social Science & Medicine,* 75(12): 2099–106.

Vrinten, C., Wardle, J. and Marlow, L.A. (2016) Cancer fear and fatalism among ethnic minority women in the United Kingdom. *British Journal of Cancer*, 114(5): 597–604.

Wallace, S., Nazroo, J. and Bécares, L. (2016) Cumulative effect of racial discrimination on the mental health of ethnic minorities in the United Kingdom. *American Journal of Public Health*, 106(7): 1294–300.

Wallen, G.R., Minniti, C.P., Krumlauf, M., Eckes, E., Allen, D., Oguhebe, A., et al. (2014) Sleep disturbance, depression and pain in adults with sickle cell disease. *BMC Psychiatry*, 14(1): 207.

Watson, J. (1988) Nursing: human science and human care. A theory of nursing. *National Nursing League Publications*, 15-2236: 1–104.

Watson, J. (2008) *Nursing: The Philosophy and Science of Caring* (rev. ed.). Boulder, CO: University Press of Colorado.

Weerasinghe, S. (2012) Inequalities in visible minority immigrant women's healthcare accessibility. *Ethnicity and Inequalities in Health and Social Care*, 5(1): 18–28.

Welsh Government (2018) *Learning Disability: Improving Lives Programme*. Available at: https://gweddill.gov.wales/docs/dhss/publications/learning-disability-improving-lives-programme.pdf (accessed 28 September 2019).

Werner, S. and Shulman, C. (2015) Does type of disability make a difference in affiliate stigma among family caregivers of individuals with autism, intellectual disability or physical disability? *Journal of Intellectual Disability Research*, 59(3): 272–83.

Wessendorf, S. (2014) *Commonplace Diversity: Social Relations in a Super-Diverse Context*. New York: Springer.

White, K. (2002) An Introduction to the Sociology of Health and Illness. Available at: www.nacro.org.uk/data/files/prevalence-patterns-and-possibilities1051.pdf (accessed 2 May 2017).

Whyte, B. (2018) Life expectancy in Calton – no longer 54. Glasgow Centre for Population Health. *The Lancet*. 388(10042): 401–11.

Wilkins, A., Mailoo, V.J. and Kularatne, U. (2010) Care of the older person: a Buddhist perspective. *Nursing and Residential Care*, 12(6): 295–7.

Williamson, M. and Harrison, L. (2010) Providing culturally appropriate care: a literature review. *International Journal of Nursing Studies*, 47: 761–9.

Wolf, M.S., Williams, M.V., Parker, R.M., Parikh, N.S., Nowlan, A.W. and Baker, D.W. (2007) Patients' shame and attitudes toward discussing the results of literacy screening. *Journal of Health Communication: International Perspectives*, 12(8): 721–32.

World Health Organization (WHO) (1948) *WHO Constitution*. Available at: www.who.int/about/who-we-are/constitution (accessed 29 September 2019).

World Health Organization (WHO) (2008a) *A Global Approach to Health Equity*. Available at: www.who.int/social_determinants/final_report/csdh_finalreport_2008_part1.pdf (accessed 3 September 2019).

World Health Organization (WHO) (2008b) *Closing the Gap in a Generation: Health Equity through Action on the Social Determinants of Health.* Available at: http://apps.who.int/iris/bitstream/handle/10665/43943/9789241563703_eng.pdf?sequence=1 (accessed 29 August 2019).

World Health Organization (WHO) (2008c) *Social Determinants of Health: Key Concepts.* Available at: www.who.int/social_determinants/thecommission/finalreport/key_concepts/en/ (accessed 6 October 2019).

World Health Organization (WHO) (2011) *Behind the 'Glasgow Effect'.* Available at: www.who.int/bulletin/volumes/89/10/11-021011/en/ (accessed 29 August 2019).

World Health Organization (WHO) (2013) *Health Literacy: The Solid Facts.* Available at: www.euro.who.int/__data/assets/pdf_file/0008/190655/e96854.pdf (accessed 28 April 2018).

World Health Organization (WHO) (2018a) *Noncommunicable Diseases: Key Facts.* Available at: www.who.int/news-room/fact-sheetds/detail/noncommunicable-diseases (accessed 3 September 2019).

World Health Organization (WHO) (2018b) *Tuberculosis: Key Facts.* Available at: www.who.int/news-room/fact-sheets/detail/tuberculosis (accessed 3 September 2019).

World Health Organization (WHO) (n.d. a) *Health Topics: Epidemiology.* Available at: www.who.int/topics/epidemiology/en/ (accessed 3 September 2019).

World Health Organization (WHO) (n.d. b) *Health Topics: Health Policy.* Available at: www.who.int/topics/health_policy/en/ (accessed 4 September 2019).

Wylie, K., Knudson, G., Khan, S.I., Bonierbale, M., Watanyusakul, S. and Baral, S. (2016) Serving transgender people: clinical care considerations and service delivery models in transgender health. *The Lancet*, 388(10042): 401–41.

Zenner, D., Abubakar, I., Conti, S., Gupta, R., Yin, Z., Kall, M., et al. (2015) Impact of TB on the survival of people living with HIV infection in England, Wales and Northern Ireland. *Thorax*, 70(6): 566–73.

Index

ability 59; *see also* disability
abuse of older people 146–7
access to services 33, 40, 55, 84, 94, 138
accountability 6, 21, 43, 69, 71, 154
acculturation 107–8, 122–3
Acheson, D. 130
activities of living (AL) 76–7
advocacy 18
age 59, 108, 152; awareness of your own 99;
    critical approach 104; cultural competency 106;
    Equality Act 10, 37; labels 107; NHS statement
    on 95–6; reflection on 97; social determinants of
    health 150; subcultures 72
alcohol 25–6, 34, 131, 135, 136, 151
alpha thalassemia 39
Alslman, E.T. 23
alternative medicine 72
anti-Semitism 10
antimicrobial resistance 131
anxiety 52–3, 63, 120, 166
Argyle, M. 58
Ashley, W. 62
assessment 69, 94–111; activities of living 77;
    challenges in planning care 107–8;
    communication 56; complexity of 97–8;
    cultural awareness 98–101; cultural competency
    105–7; equality and inclusivity 103–4; key points
    108; LEARN model 83; relevance of patients'
    beliefs 102–3
asylum seekers 8, 9, 35–6, 131, 140, 166

Bach, S. 59
Bachmann, C.L. 25
Baggott, R. 145
Baines, S. 27
BAME *see* black, Asian and minority ethnic groups
Barrett, D. 76
beliefs: acculturation 122; awareness of your own 46,
    72, 85, 97, 99, 108, 113; communication
    hindered by 49; cultural awareness 98, 99–101,
    104, 106, 109; cultural competency 77, 106;
    cultural differences 108; definition of culture 70;
    Equality Act 115; imposing religious beliefs 113;
    NHS statement on 95–6; person-centred care
    53, 103; reflection on 97; relevance of patients'
    beliefs to assessment 102–3; sensitivity to 122;
    traditional 110
Bell, R. 35
Bennett, David 164–5
Bettancourt, J.R. 74–5

bias 31, 59, 101, 106; cultural 85; paralanguage 62;
    unconscious 16–17, 18, 29, 144
biomedical model 71, 102, 103, 166
black, Asian and minority ethnic (BAME)
    groups 8, 9, 14, 18, 32–3, 152; breast cancer
    screening 28; cancer screening 143–4;
    dementia 166; demographic changes 133;
    diabetes 134, 137; inequalities 35–6; lack of NHS
    staff diversity 165–6; life expectancy 36; mental
    health 55, 120, 155, 156–61, 162, 168–9; racial
    discrimination 12; religion 121; women 16, 38;
    see also ethnicity; race
blood transfusions 78, 90
body language *see* non-verbal communication
Bowler, B. 86
Bradby, H. 8
Braedel-Kühner, C. 11
Brand, T. 8
breast cancer 28, 38
Bristowe, K. 25
Bucknor-Ferron, P. 17
Burnham, J. 58

Caldeira, S. 114
Campinha-Bacote, Josepha 75, 79–80
cancer 28, 38, 131, 133, 136, 143–5, 152
Caraher, M. 145
care: communication 46; inclusive 102; NMC
    Standards 95; quality of 84; 6 Cs 7; social context
    168; spiritual 117–18, 126, 127
care planning 69, 94, 96, 97, 112; challenges 107–8;
    cultural awareness 98; person-centred 104–5
Cartwright, Samuel 160
cervical screening 38, 144–5, 152
Chaffee, M.W. 146
chaplaincy 116, 126
children: communication with 48–9; cultural
    awareness 99; Marmot Review 139; public
    health 131; safeguarding 66
Chopra, D. 115
Christianity 14, 114, 118–19, 121, 123, 126
chronic obstructive pulmonary disease (COPD)
    132, 133, 136
Clarke, J. 118
Clarridge, A. 113
class 46, 59, 150
co-production 168
Codjoe, L. 120, 121, 122
collaboration 2, 64; communication 46; cultural safety
    84–5; cultural sensitivity 81; LEARN model 83

commissioning 168–9
commitment 7, 46
communicable diseases 134, 135–6
communication 2, 31, 43–68, 89, 126;
    barriers to 62–4; clear and open 108;
    communication skills 4, 97; cultural sensitivity 81;
    definition of 52, 55; interpersonal 59;
    interpreters 58, 63, 170; intrapersonal 61–2;
    learning disabilities 27; news of a death 123–4;
    non-verbal 52, 55–6, 58, 59, 60–1, 66, 77;
    self-awareness 46–51; 6 Cs 7; transactional
    communication model 52, 55–6;
    verbal 55–6, 57–8, 77
communities of interest 168
community public health nurses 131
compassion 2, 82, 84; chaplaincy 126;
    communication 46, 64; end-of-life care 125;
    6 Cs 7; spiritual care 118
Compassion in Practice 2, 46, 57, 74
competence 7, 46, 73–4, 88–9; *see also* cultural
    competency
confidentiality 66
consent 27
consistency 7
cooperation 2, 46
coordination of care 6, 21, 95, 129
Coulter, A. 50
courage 7, 46
Crenshaw, K. 15
critical approach 104
critical thinking 4
Cromarty, H. 25
Culley, Lorraine 11
cultural awareness 88, 98–101, 106, 109; assessment
    104, 108; models of cultural competence 79, 81,
    82; person-centred care 103
cultural competency 2–3, 69–93, 105–7; assessment
    108; definition of 74–5; mental health 167;
    models 78–83
cultural desire 75, 80
cultural encounter 75, 80
cultural knowledge 79, 81, 82, 103, 106, 109
cultural safety 84–5
cultural sensitivity 81, 82, 103, 106, 157; *see also*
    sensitivity
cultural skill 79–80, 106–7
culturally congruent care 77
culture 9–10, 29, 59, 85–6, 121;
    acculturation 107–8, 122–3; assessment 102, 104;
    awareness of your own 97, 99; communication
    issues 53; complexity of 70; cultural differences
    71–2; culture care 109, 110; definition of 155;
    eye contact 60; intersectionality 16; mental
    health 162, 167; religion 122; stereotyping 47;
    unconscious bias 17

Darzi, Lord 84
death 3, 123–6
dementia 131, 166
demography 24, 28, 29, 45, 133
Department of Health 23, 52
depression 38, 120–1, 163, 166, 170

diabetes 14, 65–6, 121, 136–8; Action for Diabetes 147;
    cultural awareness 100; ethnic groups 32, 33, 134,
    137–8; local differences 151;
    mental health problems 15; numbers living
    with 133; social determinants of health 150;
    tuberculosis comorbidity 135
diet 33, 90–1, 100, 110
difference 8, 10, 11, 101; *see also* diversity
dignity 82, 89, 118, 125, 157
disability 2, 152; austerity measures 148; critical
    approach 104; Equality Act 10, 37; NHS statement
    on 95–6; population data 14; reflection on 97;
    see also learning disabilities
discrimination 145, 168, 169; challenging 81, 157,
    158; due regard 38; Equality Act 37; gypsy
    Roma travellers 25, 30; homeless people 152;
    intersectionality 16; learning disabilities 12, 15,
    16, 26, 139; LGBTQ community 25–6, 30, 149;
    racial 9, 10–11, 12, 18, 25, 160, 162; stigma 29;
    tuberculosis 136
diversity 1–2, 11, 96; assessment 103–4; data on 14–15;
    definition of 8; super-diversity 8–9
drug use 25–6, 34, 120, 135, 149
due regard 38
duty of care 72, 84, 103

education 18, 40, 59; awareness of your own 99;
    cultural competency 106; health beliefs 103;
    values and beliefs 122
Emami, Azita 75
Emerson, E. 27
emotions 63
empathy 17, 60
end-of-life care 86, 124–6
epidemiology 28, 134, 135
equality 12, 64, 96; assessment 103–4; legislation 37; of
    opportunity 38
Equality Act (2010) 10, 15, 37, 38, 101, 103, 115, 158
Equality and Human Rights Commission (EHRC) 15
equity 12, 46
Errol McKellar Foundation 144
Essence of Care benchmarks 56
ethnicity 9–10, 12, 59, 101, 108, 117, 121;
    critical approach 104; cultural competency 106;
    death 123; definition of 155; definition of diversity
    8; demographic changes 133; demography 29;
    diabetes 137, 138; ethnic minority population 15;
    health conditions 22; health disparities 130–1;
    intersectionality 16; labels 107; life expectancy
    36; local differences 151, 152; mental health 120,
    155; religion 121; sickle-cell anaemia 39; social
    determinants of health 36, 150; unconscious
    bias 17; *see also* black, Asian and minority ethnic
    groups; race
Everett, J.S. 105
evidence-based care 71, 85
eye contact 60

Fernando, S. 155, 156, 161
force-feeding 70, 72
Francis Report (2013) 74, 84, 148
Fredrickson, G.M. 10–11

Garner, S. 9

gender 38, 59, 64, 108, 152; awareness of
    your own 99; critical approach 104; cultural
    competency 106; determinants of health 40;
    health beliefs 103; intersectionality 15, 16;
    labels 107; life expectancy 36; minority
    communities 166; NHS statement on 95–6;
    reflection on 97; social determinants
    of health 36, 150; *see also* women

gender reassignment 10, 37, 95–6, 97

genetics 29, 33, 40

genomics 28

Gerrish, Kate 75

Giddens, A. 72

'Glasgow effect' 34

Glen, S. 84

globalisation 107

Gooch, R. 25

Grant, A. 59

Green, E.M. 155

Greenfields, M. 24

gypsies/travellers 2, 24–5, 133; communication with
    45, 48–9; health conditions 22; health disparities
    131; inequalities 35–6; life expectancy 37; literacy
    45; mental health problems 120; poor health 15;
    population data 14; stigma 30; as unseen
    minority 157

Hall, S. 9

Haney, A.M. 121

Harrison, L. 104

Hatton, C. 27

health 22–4; BAME population 32–3; determinants
    of 33–4, 40, 131, 139, 140; gypsy Roma travellers
    24–5, 30; learning disabilities 26–7; LGBTQ
    community 25–6, 30; social determinants of 13,
    34–7, 130, 131–2, 150

Health Education England 29

Health Foundation 23, 24, 42

health improvement 139, 141–2

health literacy 44, 45–6, 53, 64–5, 80

health promotion 6, 21, 43, 94, 112, 129, 154

health protection 139, 142–3

Heaslip, V. 108

Henderson, S. 75

high blood pressure 32–3

Hinduism 100, 110, 114

HIV 135, 136

holistic care 168

Holland, L. 160

homeless people 34, 131, 133, 135, 140,
    142–3, 149, 152

homophobia 10, 30, 159

Hordern, J. 86

Human Genome Project 28

human rights 25, 96

identity 155, 167

immigrants 8, 122, 166; *see also* migrants

immunisations 142–3

inclusion health 133

income 40

inequalities 8, 9, 12–14, 150–1, 158; access to
    healthcare 138; challenging 81; difference and 10,
    11; gypsy Roma travellers 25; mental health care
    169; policy 146, 148; Public Health Outcomes
    Framework 139; racial discrimination 160; social
    determinants of health 13, 34, 35–6, 130, 150

influenza 142–3

information provision 84

institutionalised racism 159, 165

interpersonal communication 59

interpreters 58, 63, 170

intersectionality 15–16, 38

intrapersonal communication 61–2

Islam 16, 91, 114, 123

Islamophobia 10, 18

Jamieson, S. 114, 117–18

Jhita, T. 33

Jirwe, Maria 75

Johl, N. 166

Jorm, A.F. 53–4

Judaism 16, 86, 90–1, 114

Keating, F. 156

Kirkbride, J.B. 155

Klonoff, E.A. 122

Knapp, M. 162

labels 107

Landrine, H. 122

language: interpreters 58–9, 63, 170; language barriers
    50, 55, 57, 63–4, 109; linguistic needs 50, 53;
    misunderstandings 163, 170; paralanguage 62

LanguageLine 58

Larsson, P. 162

Lassiter, J.M. 120–1

Latif, Z. 166

leadership 4, 131, 149

LEARN model 80, 83

learning disabilities 2, 19, 26–7, 117, 121, 133, 139;
    cervical screening 144–5, 152; communication
    47–8, 65; definition of diversity 8; discrimination
    12; end-of-life care 124–5, 126; health conditions
    22; health disparities 131; inequalities 35–6;
    intersectionality 16; Learning Disabilities
    Mortality Review 144; life expectancy 36, 37;
    mental health problems 120; mortality 15;
    population data 14; social determinants of health
    150; stigma 30; *see also* disability

Ledger, P. 86

left-handedness 80

legislation 10, 15, 37, 38, 101, 103, 115, 145–6, 158

Leininger, Madeleine 75

lesbian, gay, bisexual, transgender and queer (LGBTQ)
    community 2, 25–6, 101, 117; cervical screening
    145; definition of diversity 8; demographic changes
    133; family 109; health conditions 22; health
    disparities 131; intersectionality 16; lesbian and
    bisexual women 15; marginalisation 12; mental
    health problems 120; population data 14; religion
    and spirituality 120–1; smoking 149, 152–3; stigma
    30; subcultures 72; *see also* sexual orientation

Lexico 52, 74, 84
life expectancy 27, 34, 36–7, 96, 130, 132–3, 139
linguistic diversity 163
linguistic needs 50, 53
listening 60, 83, 97, 103
literacy 45
Luchenski, S. 133

Marmot Review 12–13, 19, 35–6, 139, 148
marriage/civil partnership 37, 95–6
maternity 37, 95–6
McCarthy, J. 56
McCullough, S. 146
McDonald, A. 50
McManus, S. 155
McSherry, W. 114, 117–18
Memon, A. 55
Mencap 15, 19
Mendes, A. 119
mental health 2, 3, 34, 154–71; definition of
      diversity 8; intersectionality 16; learning
      disabilities 26; LGBTQ community 25–6, 120, 149;
      life expectancy 37; National Service Framework
      for Mental Health 54–5; paralanguage 62; physical
      illness 15; policy 147; religion 119–23; social
      determinants of health 36
Mental Health Foundation 120
mental health literacy (MHL) 53–4, 66
Metzl, J. 159
migrants 35–6, 131, 135; *see also* immigrants
minority populations 156, 166; *see also* black, Asian and
      minority ethnic groups
Morgan, C. 161
Müller, A. 11
multidisciplinary teams (MDTs) 26, 39, 46
Murray, R.B. 115

National Health Service (NHS) 95–6, 130; equity and
      equality 12, 46; gypsy Roma travellers 24–5, 30;
      lack of staff diversity 165–6; learning disabilities
      27; poor communication 50, 51; quality of care
      84; religion 116; social determinants of health 35
National Institute for Health and Care Excellence
      (NICE) 14
National Literacy Trust 53
National Service Framework for Mental Health 54–5
Nelson, T.D. 10
NHS *see* National Health Service
NHS Scotland Chaplaincy Services 116, 127
NMC *see* Nursing and Midwifery Council
NMC Standards of Proficiency for Registered Nurses
      1, 3–4, 6, 21, 43, 84, 112; assessment 94–5; cultural
      competency 69; health literacy 45; mental health 119,
      154; public health 129; respect for difference 101
non-communicable diseases (NCDs) 132, 133, 134, 136–7
non-verbal communication 52, 55–6, 58, 59, 60–1, 66, 77
Norouzinia, R. 57
Nursing and Midwifery Council (NMC) 1; code
      of conduct 25, 46, 72, 85, 101, 116, 125, 157;
      communication 57; community public health
      nurses 131; competence 73, 74; person-centred
      care 53; safeguarding 66; spirituality 86

nursing models 76–8
Nutbeam, D. 162
Nyatanga, B. 124, 127

obesity 131, 145–6, 147, 151
O'Connell, M.B. 85
Office for National Statistics (ONS) 7, 20
O'Hagan, K. 101
older people 101, 131, 146–7, 166
Oozageer Gunowa, N. 105
Ousey, K. 160
Owen, D. 156

pain 19, 52–3
palliative care 124–6
Papadopoulos, Irena 75, 81, 82
paralanguage 62
parents 48–9, 99
Parikh, N.S. 53
patient-centred care 16–17
Pentaris, P. 123
Perez-Bret, E. 82
person-centred care 49, 53, 84, 98, 103, 105
personalisation 168
Pesut, B. 114, 118
Pezella, A. 82
physical environment 33, 40
placements 89
policy 145–8, 150–1, 162, 163
politics 162–3
poverty 147, 148, 158, 160
pregnancy 37, 95–6
prejudice 10, 16, 29, 59, 81, 85, 97
Price, B. 62
privacy 66, 80, 118
professional barriers 63
professional nursing culture 71
Promotion of Safe and Therapeutic
      Services (PSTS) 165
prostate cancer screening 143–4
proximity 61, 65
psychosis 155, 159
public health 3, 129–53, 169
Public Health England 45, 54, 92, 131, 133, 152
Public Health Outcomes Framework (PHOF) 139
Purnell, L. 77

Qassem, T. 155
quality 83, 84–5

race 9–10, 59, 165; awareness of your own 99;
      cultural competency 106; definition of 155;
      Equality Act 10, 37; intersectionality 15; NHS
      statement on 95–6; paralanguage 62; reflection
      on 97; Runnymede Trust 42; skin colour 105;
      unconscious bias 17; *see also* black, Asian and
      minority ethnic groups; ethnicity
racial discrimination 9, 10–11, 12, 18, 25, 160, 162
racism 10–11, 158–9, 162, 165, 167; gypsy Roma
      travellers 30; as public health issue 169;
      Runnymede Trust 42; social determinants of
      health 36

Ramezani, M. 117
rapport 56, 77
Rauf, A. 166
RCN *see* Royal College of Nursing
reasonable adjustment 37
reflection 4, 61–2
refugees 9, 49–50, 140–1
Rehman, H. 156
Reimer-Kirkham, S. 114
relationships 64
religion 59, 86–8, 90–1, 108, 113–23, 126;
    acculturation 122–3; awareness of your own 99;
    critical approach 104; cultural awareness 100;
    cultural competency 106; death 123–4, 126;
    Equality Act 10, 37, 115; influence on health
    beliefs 102–3; intersectionality 16; mental health
    and 119–23; NHS statement on 95–6; population
    data 14; reflection on 97; social determinants of
    health 150; subcultures 72; *see also* spirituality
resilience 162, 168
respect 64, 80, 82, 89, 125
Richardson, B. 62
Robinson, F. 25
role modelling 47, 163
Rollock, D. 121
Roma 2, 24–5; communication with 48–9; health
    conditions 22; inequalities 35–6; life expectancy
    37; literacy 45; mental health problems 120; as
    unseen minority 157; *see also* travellers
Roper–Logan–Tierney model 76–8
Roper, N. 77, 78
Royal College of General Physicians 46
Royal College of Nursing (RCN) 25, 74, 86, 99;
    guidance on religious and spiritual care 126;
    personal beliefs 113; placements 89; policy 148;
    survey on religion 117
Runnymede Trust 42

safeguarding 66
Scadding, J. 45
schizophrenia 159, 164
self-awareness 46–51, 58, 72, 79, 106
sensitivity 2, 64, 80; communication 46, 49; cultural 81,
    82, 103, 106, 157; religious beliefs 122
sex 10, 37, 38
sexual orientation 59, 121, 152; awareness of your own
    99; critical approach 104; definition of diversity
    8; Equality Act 10, 37; NHS statement on 95–6;
    reflection on 97; *see also* lesbian, gay, bisexual,
    transgender and queer community
shame 53, 63, 121
Shulman, C. 30
sickle-cell anaemia 29, 31, 39
Sikhism 114
6 Cs 2, 7, 46, 82, 85
skin colour 105
smoking 25–6, 131, 136, 149, 151, 152–3
social determinants of health 13, 34–7, 130, 131–2, 150
social environment 33, 40
social position 104
social support 40

socio-economic status 103, 104, 106
Soft Drinks Industry Levy 130, 145–6
Solomos, J. 11
spirituality 3, 59, 86, 104, 114–23, 126, 127; *see also*
    religion
Srivastava, S.B. 71, 72, 77
stereotyping 10, 17, 47, 59, 83, 85; assessment 101, 104,
    108; care planning 107–8; cultural awareness 106;
    cultural knowledge 79; gypsy Roma travellers 30;
    paralanguage 62
stigma 29–31, 40; mental health 156, 157, 161, 162,
    166–7, 168, 169; tuberculosis 136
strengths-based model 168
stroke 32–3
Sturmberg, J. 23
subcultures 72–3
suicide 25, 120–1
super-diversity 8–9
Sutton, P.W. 72
Sweeney, S. 45

Taylor, Gina 75, 81
Taylor, S.P. 57
teamwork 4, 26, 39, 46, 129
therapeutic relationship 50, 85
Tilki, Mary 75, 81
Timmins, F. 114
touch 60–1, 65
Tran, L. 166
transactional communication model 52, 55–6
transcultural nursing 75
transgender people 25, 38
transphobia 10
travellers 2, 24–5, 133; communication with 45, 48–9;
    health conditions 22; health disparities 131;
    inequalities 35–6; literacy 45; mental health
    problems 120; poor health 15; population data
    14; stigma 30; as unseen minority 157
Truswell, D. 166
tuberculosis 131, 132, 134, 135–6, 140–1
Tuffrey-Wijne, I. 124
Twyman, L. 149

unconscious bias 16–17, 18, 29, 31, 144
underserved populations 133, 135–6, 140–1

vaccinations 87–8, 91
values: acculturation 122; awareness of your own 46,
    72, 85, 97, 108, 113; cultural awareness 104, 106,
    109; cultural competency 77, 106; definition of
    culture 70; inclusive care 102; person-centred care
    53, 103
Valuing People (2011) 48
Venkatasalu, M.R. 123
verbal communication 55–6, 57–8, 77

Watson, Jean 103
Weerasinghe, S. 160
Werner, S. 30
WHO *see* World Health Organization
Williamson, M. 104

women: austerity measures 148; breast cancer
     screening 28, 38; cervical screening 38, 144–5,
     152; inequality 38; intersectionality 15; lesbian
     and bisexual 15; life expectancy 36; minority
     populations 156, 166; violence against 147;
     see also gender

Wood, J.T. 55
World Health Organization (WHO) 12–13, 20, 23,
     34–5, 84, 134, 159

Zagaja, L. 17
Zentner, J.B. 115